楊氏太極拳大全

楊俊敏

© **UNIQUE PUBLICATIONS, INC., 1982**
All rights reserved
Printed in the United States of America
Library of Congress No.: 81-50513
ISBN: 0-86568-023-X

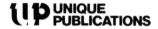

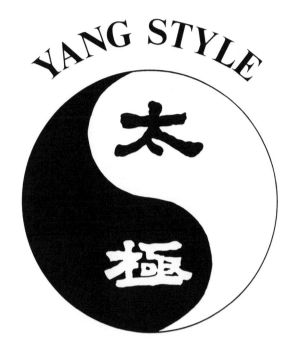

YANG STYLE

TAI CHI CHUAN

By Yang Jwing-Ming

ACKNOWLEDGEMENTS
The author wishes to thank Vidas Gvozdzius for editing this book. In addition, the author would also like to thank Cosmin Theodore and Joe Sbarounis for the time they spent in helping with the general construction of the book.

This volume is dedicated to my first Tai Chi teacher, Mr. Kao Taou, who built the foundation of my Tai Chi Chuan.

PREFACE

It is quite ironic that Tai Chi Chuan, one of the oldest pugilistic systems in China, is at once the most popular as well as misunderstood Chinese martial art that is currently practiced. Tai Chi is the most popular of the Chinese martial arts because large numbers of people practice it for health and relaxation; on the other hand, Tai Chi is misunderstood because few people realize its martial foundation. This split between practice for health and practice for defense began early in the 20th century because more people began to use it as an easy method of exercise. At the same time, fewer people were studying it as a martial art. Therefore, a book which can combine both elements, defense and health, is much needed at this time. This book, then, will attempt to bridge the gap between theory and practice so that the reader can see Tai Chi Chuan, specifically Yang's style, in its complete form. This book can thus be used by the martial Tai Chi practitioner, the beginner who is interested in starting Tai Chi as a serious discipline, and the person who is only interested in Tai Chi as a form of nonviolent exercise.

Besides delineating the martial and health theories behind Yang's style of Tai Chi Chuan, this book will also contain many other special features. First, Yang's traditional barehand sequence will be shown in its entirety with the correct breathing intervals. To show Yang's style of Tai Chi Chuan in its most complete form, it is extremely important to show the barehand form without eliminating any parts. Currently, many Tai Chi instructors have devised shortened and simplified versions which are easier to learn, but which do not promote the beneficial aspects of Tai Chi because the reduced sequence does not allow enough time and movement for full exercise and relaxation. The original sequence was devised to include enough forms to facilitate proper exercise; thus, its complete form is very important. In addition, by reducing the sequence, important martial techniques are eliminated. While Yang's original barehand sequence is relatively long, this book will provide in-depth explanations with many pictures of transient forms.

Second, in the way of martial purpose, the practical use of each Tai Chi barehand form will be shown. The martial aspect will be further extended by showing and explaining the theory and techniques of the extremely important practice of *pushing hands* (Tuei Sou). The next step in achieving martial applicability will be showing and explaining the two-man Tai Chi *fighting sequence*. With the finish of the fighting sequence, this book will have presented the full range of all the martial barehand techniques of Yang's Tai Chi Chuan.

Third, to compliment the barehand techniques of Tai Chi, this book will present the famous and elegant Tai Chi narrow blade sword sequence. Like the other aspects of this book, the martial and health aspects of the Tai Chi sword will be explained. Although mastering the Tai Chi sword in actual combat is one of the highest achievements in Chinese martial arts, taking years to master, it is important to record this high art for future generations.

A fourth feature of this book is Yang's style of Tai Chi Chuan itself. Yang's system is one of the most popular in the world. Low postures, large forms, and practical martial techniques make Yang's style one of the most beautiful and deadly martial arts in the world.

Lastly, it would help to understand the reasons for publishing this book. With the growing interest in Tai Chi Chuan many changes have occurred in its traditional forms and ideas. While change is not necessarily negative, it is vital not to abandon aspects which have been formulated and tested through hundreds of years of experience, research, and practice. By having a book grounded in traditional practice, a basis is formed for further research that starts from principles which have been found to be valid over the centuries. In this way, a newcomer or a practiced veteran can avoid many confusing changes and false concepts. Hopefully, this book will help in the continued preservation, improvement, and practice of this great art.

CONTENTS

Preface

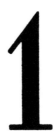

GENERAL INTRODUCTION

Background of Tai Chi

Philosophically, the major concepts of Tai Chi Chuan are rooted in Taoism. In particular, two major Taoist texts were, and are still today, important for the Tai Chi practitioner: the *Tao Te Ching* and the *I Ching*. While neither book is in any way a martial manual, both books firmly establish a way of thinking about the world which affected every aspect of Tai Chi Chuan from breathing techniques to power development.

In the *Tao Te Ching,* a book of poems reputedly written by Li Erh or Lao Tzu about the fourth century B.C., one of its major themes which has come to dominate and influence Tai Chi is the idea of Tao. As presented by Lao Tzu, Tao is the ultimate reality from which all things evolved. Therefore, the goal of life is to follow, without contention, the natural order of the manifestations of Tao, and eventually Tao itself. The emphasis on doing the natural according to the laws of the universe, versus the forced or artifical, was very important to Lao Tzu. The scholar Fung Yu-Lan has stated that, "If one understands these laws and regulates one's actions in conformity with them, one can then turn everything to one's advantage."* It is out of this basic idea that Tai Chi received its name, which means the Grand Ultimate. The basic goal inherent in the idea of Tai Chi, or the Grand Ultimate, is to return to the original source of the universe. The closer one can get to the first principle or cause, the more one completes himself. Thus, Tai Chi practitioners have taken this idea of the Grand Ultimate and have applied it to their martial system. For fighting or for health, the Tai Chi artist will follow the natural inclination of things.

From the *I Ching,* a book over two thousand years older than Lao Tzu's *Tao Te Ching,* Tai Chi martial artists took the concept of Yin and Yang. In the natural flow of events, the operating principle that drives the universe is the interplay of two polar forces—Yin and Yang. The Yin is considered the passive force while Yang is considered the active force. Between the dynamic tension of Yin and Yang, all things find their nature.

In the *I Ching* the dynamic interplay of Yin and Yang is represented by two dashed line (––, Yin) and a single dashed line (—, Yang). These lines are then arranged into groups of three (e.g., ☳) and six (e.g., ☷). Traditionally, the discovery of the trigrams, of which there are eight, is attributed to Fu Hsi around the period of 2852-2738 B.C. Later, King Wen combined the trigrams into hexagrams, of which there are sixty-four. Because Yin and Yang are fundamental principles, the eight trigrams and sixty-four hexagrams can be used to understand the mysteries of nature. These representations of Yin and Yang can then be used to predict everything from the birth of a child to the fate of a nation.

From the important and fundamental trigrams, Tai Chi Chuan evolved its basic martial strategies. First, by looking at the arrangement of the Ba Kua, the eight original trigrams, two systems can be separated (Figure 1): the trigrams that are perpendicular to the center, and those that are diagonal to the center. For easier reference, these positions can be represented by a compass system as N, NE, E, SE, S, SW, W, and NW. The early Tai Chi practitioners came to believe that the eight trigrams represented all the basic directions to which a martial artist could move during a fight.

Along with representing the eight fundamental directions of movement, the trigrams correspond to the eight basic techniques of Tai Chi. Each of the eight techniques was assigned a direction and a trigram to describe its fundamental nature, as shown in Figure 1. For example, the technique of Ward-Off is composed of three lines which are symbolic of the Yang principle; therefore, this particular technique contains extreme energy and is used with a great explosions of power. The three Yang lines indicate

8   *Fung Yu-Lan, *A Short History of Chinese Philosophy,* (New York: MacMillan), 1961, p. 65.

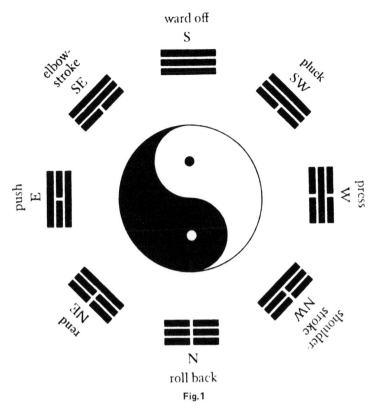

ward off
S

elbow-stroke
SE

pluck
SW

push
E

press
W

rend
NE

shoulder-stroke
NW

N

roll back

Fig.1

that its explosiveness requires exhalation to bring out the full power of the practitioner. On the other hand, the technique of Roll Back contains three Yin lines; therefore, this technique is purely defensive and requires inhalation; it absorbs rather than attacks. A technique such as Push is a mixture of offensive and defensive, although the offensive will dominate because there are two Yang lines to the one Yin line.

In addition to the various directions of movement, the Tai Chi theorists added active movements which represented the five basic elements which compose the universe: Metal (Gin), Wood (Moo), Water (Sui), Fire (Fou), and Earth (Tu). The five elements are called the Wu Shing and correspond to the movements of *advance, retreat, dodge and beware of the left, dodge and beware of the right,* and *holding the center.* Taken together, these thirteen elements are formally known as the Thirteen Postures (Shih Shan Shih). The Thirteen Postures are one of the foundation stones for Tai Chi as a martial art. In fact, many people have called the art Shih Shan Shih in reference to its fundamental principles.

The *I Ching* also influenced Tai Chi Chuan in other different and subtle ways. For example, in terms of the overall style, Tai Chi has two types of meditation that are considered Yin and Yang: conventional sitting meditation and the moving meditation of the Tai Chi sequence. Taken together, both are needed to fully develop the Yin and Yang aspects of health and martial defense. On a smaller scale, the act of breathing has been broken down into a Yin and Yang relationship: inhaling is Yin and exhaling is Yang.

With this short introduction, the reader can hopefully have a general idea of the philosophical background of Tai Chi. For a more complete discussion on the *Tao Te Ching* and the *I Ching,* the reader can consult many good scholarly books on this subject. Once the reader has fully acquainted himself with the principles of the two books, he can more clearly see the underlying general theory behind Tai Chi Chuan.

History of Yang's Tai Chi Chuan

Traditionally, Tai Chi Chuan has been known by four different names according to personal preferences and local customs. These names are Tai Chi Chuan, Shih Shan Shih, Mei Chuan, and Chang Chuan. The first two names were discussed earlier in this chapter. Tai Chi was called Mei Chuan because the phrase means "soft sequence," and referred to the relaxed and gentle way in which the forms were performed. Chang Chuan, the last name used to refer to Tai Chi, means "long sequence." The Tai Chi barehand sequence, in comparison to those of other martial styles, takes much longer to perform while also containing a larger number of techniques—thus, the long sequence. (There is also a Shao Lin style called Chang Chuan, but in this case the phrase means Long Fist, referring to the styles of long range fighting maneuvers.)

From a more factual historical perspective, the early development of Tai Chi Chuan is rather vague. In general, many people credit Chang Shan-Fon with originating Tai Chi in the thirteenth century A.D. (Sung Dynasty), when he combined martial techniques based on the movements of the snake and white crane with *internal power*. (Internal power is the ability to use *Chi*. See next chapter for a definition of Chi. The opposite of internal power is *external power*, which is strength generated solely by the muscles. External power is not considered as potent as internal power because it is limited, while the internal power is not.) While the martial artists of the famous Shao Lin Temple were using the internal power methods of an Indian Buddhist named Da Mo, Chang Shan-Fon was the first to use a style which fully incorporated internal power with fighting techniques. Although Chang Shan-Fon is credited with being one of the early founders of Tai Chi, the style may have developed within a division of the Shao Lin Temple in Wu Dan Mountain. (The main Shaolin Temple was located in Huo Nan province.) When Chang was alive, the Shao Lin Temple system of martial arts had already been in existence for 800 years. Among the Temples were those that continued to develop the internal power methods of Da Mo. Quite conceivably, Tai Chi may have been a special division of the Shao Lin Temple.

It is not until the middle of the eighteenth century that the history becomes more clear and precise. During that time, a man named Chen Chang Shen was teaching Tai Chi to his relatives and a few select outsiders. Traditionally, the teaching of many martial systems was tightly restricted to relatives and people with the same surname. Very rarely were non-related people allowed to learn the deeper aspects of a family martial art. Chen Chang Shen was teaching his particular family style of Tai Chi Chuan in Chen Jar Gao, in the province of Huo Nan.

It happened that at this time a man named Yang Lu Shann (1780-1873) wanted to learn Tai Chi. Because Yang Lu Shann wasn't a member of Chen Chang Shen's family, he had difficulty in gaining entrance; but, Yang Lu Shann did eventually gain entrance into the family as a servant. As a member of the family household, Chen Chang Shen taught Yang Lu Shann Tai Chi, but only its surface knowledge. For a long time Yang Lu Shan was disappointed that he was not learning the key martial aspects of the system. Nevertheless, he faithfully and diligently practiced what he was taught.

Yang Lu Shann's progress in mastering Tai Chi was painfully slow until one fateful night. On that particular night, at midnight, Yang Lu Shann was awakened by faint shouting sounds that came from a distance. Getting up to investigate the sounds, he followed the shouts until he came upon Chen Chang Shen with a group of students. Yang Lu Shann carefully hid himself and observed all the martial secrets which Chen was teaching. Among the things which Yang Lu Shann learned were the Hun and Ha method method of shouting for the generation of power. Up to this time, Yang Lu Shann could not use his power for martial purposes. In addition, Yang Lu Shann learned how to apply all the techniques from the barehand sequence. Although Chen Chang Shen taught Yang Lu Shann the forms of Tai Chi, he did not teach him their martial applications. Later that day, Yang Lu Shann went off by himself to practice the things which he observed. From that time, Yang Lu Shann secretly observed the midnight sessions and then practiced everything he had seen.

One day it happened that Chen Chang Shen asked Yang Lu Shann to spar with the students who practiced secretly each midnight. To Chen Chang Shen's surprise, not even his best students could overcome Yang Lu Shann. From that moment Chen Chang Shen formally accepted Yang Lu Shann as a student; Yang Lu Shann was, from that point, taught the family style in earnest.

Eventually, Yang Lu Shann left Huo Nan for Peking, where he taught his three sons and a number of other pupils. His oldest son died quite young, but his other two offspring continued to study and master the style which their father learned from Chen Chang Shen. From the two remaining sons, Tai Chi was to branch itself into distinctive styles while gaining wide popularity for the system as a whole.

First, Yang Pan Huo (1837-1890) the second son, taught the style to a number of people including Wu Chun Yu. Wu Chun Yu then taught his son Wu Chien Chun (Figure 2). Wu Chien Chun later modified the style and founded the Wu style of Tai Chi Chuan. Wu's style is especially popular in Hong Kong, Singapore, and Malaysia.

The third son, Yang Chien Huo (1842-1916) (Figure 3), was to become extremely important because it was his third son, Yang Chen Fu (1883-1935) (Figure 4), who formed the distinctive characteristics of what is now known as Yang's style of Tai Chi. Until Yang Chen Fu, the Yang family had essentially taught the style of Chen Chang Shen. It wasn't until Yang Chen Fu added his own ideas and modifications that Yang's style was truly born. As a point of information, Chen Chang Shen's style, known quite naturally as Chen's style of Tai Chi, still continues to be practiced today.

Although Yang Chen Fu initiated Yang's style, he began to study and practice Tai Chi in his late teens; up to that point he resisted his father's attempts to teach him Tai Chi. But when Yang Chen Fu's father died, he became extremely interested in Tai Chi and practiced it until he was very proficient.

Among Yang Chen Fu's other achievements was the fact that he was the first person in his family

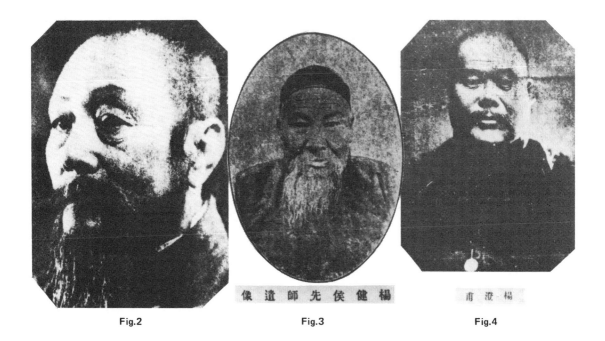

像 遺 師 先 侯 健 楊

甫 澄 楊

Fig.2   Fig.3   Fig.4

circle to spread Tai Chi beyond its original confines. Yang Chen Fu was the great popularizer of Tai Chi. Today, the practitioners of the Chen, Wu, and Yang styles of Tai Chi Chuan can be found everywhere. Although many relatives of the first developers are still alive and practicing their forefather's systems, each style has become internationally known and practiced.

The Range of Tai Chi

Tai Chi Chuan, like most complete martial systems, contains a variety of aspects which must be studied and practiced over time in order to be mastered. First, Tai Chi Chuan has theories and training techniques for two major divisions within the style: still or sitting meditation and moving meditation. Many people who practice Tai Chi do not realize that meditation is an extremely important and integral part of martial training. While many martial styles contain meditation techniques, in the majority of cases, they only serve as a calming or relaxing device. For example, one may practice and become proficient in such Shao Lin styles as Praying Mantis, Long Fist, and Eagle Claw without meditating on a constant day-to-day basis. But in Tai Chi, one cannot achieve martial proficiency without practicing sitting meditation. Meditation and its relationship to Tai Chi will be treated in the next chapter.

To compliment still meditation, Tai Chi practitioners have developed a system of moving meditation which is the basis for all their martial techniques. First, the student learns the proper method of breathing. Next, he will combine the breathing techniques with simple martial forms which are practiced in slow motion. After achieving proficiency and smoothness in breathing and form, the student will begin to learn the Tai Chi barehand sequence for the next two to three years. This sequence is the basis for all the martial techniques in the style.

While the student is learning the Tai Chi barehand sequence, he will also start the practice of pushing hands. Pushing hands practice is extremely vital to the style because it forms the basis for all free fighting. In pushing hands practice, the student learns how to dissolve, neutralize, and counterattack an opponent's offensive actions. When pushing hands is first begun, it is done very slowly so that the student will learn how to coordinate his breathing with the martial technique. From the third to fifth year, after the student has learned to coordinate breathing with technique, he will practice pushing hands with the goal of developing the ability to use his Chi for defense and attack. By the third year, the student should have cultivated enough Chi to serve this purpose.

The next stage, in the development of Tai Chi free fighting, usually after the fifth year of practice, is learning the two-man fighting sequence. In the fighting sequence two students engage in combat against each other by using prearranged techniques. The fighting sequence is first done slowly so that the practitioners will be able to coordinate the techniques with the circulation of Chi. Later, the students go on to use more power. The fighting sequence must be practiced for about five years to insure the correct use of internal power with martial technique. As a result, when the students perform the fighting sequence, they are engaged in an actual fight. The last stage is to engage in spontaneous and unrestricted free fighting.

11

To reach the final stage of proficient free fighting usually takes about ten years of practice. While many of the forms are simple, actual proficiency takes years to develop. Among other things, the student must be able to coordinate all his techniques, whether performed slowly or quickly, with the proper breathing series, to be able to dissolve and neutralize powerful attacks by using a minimum of exertion, and to be able to generate internal, or Chi, power at will. Only years of dedicated practice can achieve these results.

In terms of weapons, Tai Chi Chuan uses only a few: wide blade sword, narrow blade sword, rod, and spear. This contrasts with the Shao Lin styles, which have a wider variety of weapons. After the first three years, the student will learn the wide blade sword because this particular weapon can be used without the possession of great internal power. In the first three years of training the student will not have developed enough internal power to be effectively used in coordination with a weapon for martial purposes. But with a wide blade sword, external (muscle) power can be used as its power source.

After the tenth year, the Tai Chi practitioner will begin the study and practice of the narrow blade sword, the king of the short weapons. The narrow blade sword has traditionally been the principal weapon used by the internal divisions. Before beginning the Tai Chi sword, the practitioner must already possess internal power and extensive experience as a martial artist. This prerequisite is necessary because the Tai Chi sword, to be correctly used, requires internal power, smoothness in motion, and the ability to neutralize an opponent's power. Usually, proficiency in the narrow blade sword requires two to three years of practice. The stages leading to mastery are similar to those of barehand fighting: slow motion sequence, fighting forms of sword against sword, and then free fighting. When a person masters the Tai Chi sword, he will have one of the most respected skills in the martial arts world.

While the techniques of the narrow blade sword are being studied, the Tai Chi martial artist will also go on to study and practice the use of the rod and/or spear. With these weapons the Tai Chi practitioner will have both long range and short range fighting tools. Like the narrow blade sword, mastery of the rod and spear require that the martial artist have considerable skills beforehand. Very few individuals have gone on to master the extremely difficult techniques of rod and spear.

In summary, this rough outline of Tai Chi Chuan as a martial art shows that as a system of self-defense, Tai Chi encompasses a variety of aspects, including everything from still meditation to fast motion fighting. While learning the principles of Tai Chi takes relatively little time, the actual mastery of these principles will take years. For this reason, it is said that after eighteen years of practicing Tai Chi one can only claim a small achievement.

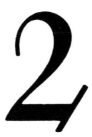

PRINCIPLES OF TAI CHI CHUAN

Chi and Chi Circulation

To understand why Tai Chi Chuan is effective as an exercise and as a powerful system of self-defense, one must understand the concept of Chi. The word itself can mean "breath," but a more accurate term is "vital energy." The best way to come to a functional definition of Chi is to compare it to the blood and the circulatory system.

Blood can be, in a manner, considered an all pervasive liquid energy which circulates through the body giving vital nourishment to every cell. The system which carries this liquid energy pervades every part of the body by means of an extensive network of veins and arteries. Any major disruption in this system may cause a person to die by either stoppage or loss of blood. For example, if a person receives a major cut, the body will quickly lose its liquid energy, causing shock or death. Likewise, a person with a blocked artery, such as a thrombosis, will also be adversely affected.

Chi, by comparison and metaphor, is an electrical kind of energy which nourishes the body on its own particular level. Chi, like blood, is a form of energy which everybody needs to exist. But even more than our need for blood is our need to have life-sustaining Chi. Chi is the energetic foundation of all life.

Like blood, Chi must travel throughout the body to nourish and maintain life. The conducting pathway for Chi is the nervous system, a system as extensive as the circulatory system. Any time that the nervous system is distrupted, as in polio or spine injuries, the Chi cannot effectively spread its beneficial energy. When the flow of Chi is stopped in any way, the individual will become ill according to the degree that Chi is hindered.

In the nervous system itself, Chi will follow certain main circuits on a cyclical basis. The cycles themselves follow natural events such as the solar day, lunar month, season, and year. This is in contrast to the circulation of blood, which flows in a constant and relatively unchanging cycle. Through hundreds of years of investigation, there have been found to be fourteen such main pathways through which Chi travels. These pathways are the twelve meridians and two vessels of acupuncture. Chi travels to every part of the body through the meridians and vessels.

According to acupuncture theory, every meridian (including the vessels whose purpose is to help overall functioning) is connected to a certain internal organ. When the Chi is flowing smoothly through the meridian, the internal organ functions well. But if the Chi flow is hindered in some way, the internal organ will not function as it should. Thus, keeping the flow of Chi unrestricted through the meridians and vessels is of vital importance for health.

When an organ starts to function improperly because of an inadequate flow of Chi, the acupuncturtist will insert a needle into a certain point on the specific meridian in order to readjust the circulation of Chi. These specific points on the meridian are stimulated in order to readjust the circulation of Chi. These specific points on the meridian are known as *cavities*, or more generally, acupuncture points. There are roughly 700 acupuncture points that are used to alter the flow of Chi for improved health.

Tai Chi Chuan and Chi Circulation

Because Tai Chi martial artists have developed their system so that it is intimately connected with the smooth circulation of Chi, the practice of this art form will lead to better health. Tai Chi, then, improves health mainly by allowing Chi to flow more actively and fluidly through the body. In addition to improved Chi circulation, the practice of Tai Chi will make blood circulation more efficient. Overall, Tai Chi allows both liquid and electric energies better and smoother flow.

One of the major ways that Tai Chi helps the individual is by its capacity to increase the local circulation (non-meridian) of Chi, especially in the extremities. When an individual does the Tai Chi sequence in a relaxed manner, the muscles around the veins, arteries, and nerves will be relaxed, allowing the Chi to distribute itself more evenly and to flow more easily in those particular areas. By improving the local circulation of Chi, less stress is put on the internal organs. Local circulation is one reason why the skin of Tai Chi practitioners is so healthy; the charge over the skin is always evenly spread.

In addition to achieving local circulation, the internal organs of an individual will be exercised because of the deep breathing which the slow motion Tai Chi sequence requires. During deep breathing, the muscles controlling the inhalation and exhalation process are required to move very low in the abdomen. This low movement exercises the internal organs in the entire abdominal region. Without deep breathing, stimulation of the organs is not possible. This is why Tai Chi is superior to many other forms of exercise which only, in most cases, violently exercise the external muscles. As an example, jogging strains the leg and lung muscles while doing relatively little for the liver, kidney, etc. Without deep breathing, Tai Chi cannot effectively improve the internal organs.

Through the combined effects of local circulation and deep breathing, Tai Chi practitioners have found that the slow motion barehand sequence can cure or help alleviate a variety of disorders. Generally, any disorder which involves the internal organs can be cured. Such dysfunctions as ulcers, hernias, high blood pressure, lung disorders, heart trouble, and tuberculosis are remedied through the practice of Tai Chi. Some of these ailments can be cured in less than a year. In addition, Tai Chi has been found helpful in alleviating arthritis, chronic headaches, and nervous conditions.

The second way that Tai Chi improves health is by making the Chi flow more smoothly through the meridians and vessels themselves. Making the Chi flow through, essentially, the whole body is also the foundation for using Tai Chi as a martial art; this aspect will be treated later. But making the Chi run more efficiently through the meridians and vessels will require more than just a calm and relaxed state; it will require either meditation and/or several years of concentrated practice of the slow motion of the Tai Chi sequence.

In meditation the primary purpose is to make the Chi flow at will through the governing (Yang) and conception (Yin) vessels in an enclosed circular pattern. This particular path is called Shao Chou Tien or Small Circulation. This cycle will run in a complete circle around the centerline on the front and back sides of the head and torso. Once the Chi can be circulated at will following the governing and conception vessels, the Chi can then be passed into the arms and legs, thus achieving Da Chou Tien or "Grand Circulation." When the Chi flows into the arms and legs from the Small Circulation, the Chi will spread into all the meridians, thereby benefiting health. The detailed theory of achieving Chi circulation through meditation will be covered in the next section.

The second method to increase Chi flow through the meridians and vessels is by doing the slow motion Tai Chi sequence for several years. Essentially, after several years of consistent practice, the Tai Chi practitioner can achieve Small Circulation by concentrating on this task. Once the Small Circulation has been obtained, the Chi can be made to spread into the arms and legs to achieve Grand Circulation. While meditation will be discussed in this chapter, the detailed aspects of the Tai Chi sequence will be shown and explained in Chapter 3.

Turning to the self-defense aspects of Tai Chi, the achievement of the Small and Grand Circulations is required during the course of training. A person cannot effectively use Tai Chi as a martial system by merely restricting himself to practicing the slow motion sequence. The martial power which the Tai Chi practitioner uses comes from the Chi that is originally developed along the path of the Small Circulation. The Tai Chi martial artist will train in special methods so that his Chi can be applied and directed into the arms and legs instantaneously with enormous power. The power generated from the Chi is then coordinated with martial forms for fighting.

In review, the main point in developing Tai Chi as a martial art and as an exercise lies in achieving a smooth circulation of Chi to every part of the body. For the person interested in Tai Chi as an exercise, achieving local circulation while deep breathing to stimulate the internal organs is enough to obtain beneficial results for health. But for the Tai Chi martial artist, the process must be extended to where the potential of Chi is trained for self-defense. Because of this extended purpose, the Tai Chi martial artist must practice his art at least ten years before he can achieve proficiency.

Meditation
Breathing

Fundamentally, the first and most important step for effective meditation is proper breathing. Basically, there are two systems which can be used during meditation: Taoist and Buddhist. Both systems are equally effective, but because Tai Chi uses the Taoist method, it will be described in detail. The interested reader can easily find many good books describing Buddhist meditation and breathing. Before the practitioner attempts meditation, he should read this whole section thoroughly to be aware of all the major points of meditation.

Taoist breathing, sometimes known as reverse breathing, is the very first step in preparing the Chi for circulation; therefore, its proper development is crucial. In Taoist breathing, the normal movement of the lower abdomen is reversed during inhalation and exhalation. When using the Taoist method, the area below the navel is sucked in during inhalation; in contrast, the Buddhist method requires that this area expand during inhalation. While inhaling, the air is slowly brought in as a thin column though the nose. Inhalation must be smooth and easy.

Once the lung is adequately filled with air, the practitioner starts gently to exhale. One must never hold the breath or force the process of inhalation or exhalation. In Tai Chi, inhalation is considered Yin and exhalation is considered Yang. They must operate like the Yin/Yang circle in Figure 1 of Chapter 1; inhalation and exhalation must run into each other smoothly and effortlessly in a fluid circular motion. As the exhalation process is occuring, the pubic region begins to lower and expand itself at a point two inches below the navel. This important point, called the Dan Tien, is the area in which the Chi will be produced and accumulated in order to start the Small Circulation. Because of this, the muscles around the Dan Tien must be trained so that they can sufficiently contract and expand while the individual inhales and exhales. At first, expanding the Dan Tien during exhalation may be difficult; but with practice, the muscles can be trained to accommodate lower expansion. One must not force the Dan Tien to expand. Instead, the practitioner should gently expand until success is achieved. As with inhalation, he should exhale smoothly and easily.

This whole process of aspiration and expiration can also be referred to as deep breathing, not because the breathing is heavy, but because the inhalation and exhalation work the lungs to near capacity. While many people who engage in strenuous exercise may breathe hard, they do not necessarily breathe deeply. While deep breathing is occuring, the internal organs vibrate to the rhythm of the breaths; the vibration of the organs stimulates or exercises them. For this reason, many benefits can be derived. The organs would not receive this type of internal exercise without deep breathing. It can be seen that many forms of violent exercise only condition the external muscles, while doing very little for the vital organs.

In addition, Taoist inhalation and exhalation is thought particularly beneficial because it imitates the breathing of an infant. Small babies breath naturally and smoothly while expanding their Dan Tien to exhale and withdrawing their Dan Tien to inhale. The Taoist and the Tai Chi practitioners, then, attempt to go back to the state of infancy when the body was full of circulating purified Chi and natural breath. Deep breathing in coordination with the contraction and expansion of the Dan Tien is a return to a healthy primal state.

The Taoist method of breathing is also the system that is used when an individual practices the Tai Chi sequence. Everything that has been said about Taoist breathing is applicable to the barehand and weapon sequences. By constant practice this method of breathing can be done without thought or strain. To practice the Taoist method of breathing, Chapter 3 has several fundamental forms which are used for this purpose.

Meditation and Chi Circulation

Once the Tai Chi practitioner can breathe adequately according to the Taoist method, he may commence sitting meditation to begin the process of Chi circulation. (For the practical aspects of meditation such as correct posture, placement of hands, tongue, etc., refer to the next section.) When the practitioner starts meditation, his first goal should be to achieve a calm mind while concentrating on deep breathing. The individual should perform a kind of self-hyponsis, inducing himself into a semi-sleeping state. The meditator should stay at this stage until he can, with no effort, expand and withdraw his Dan Tien while breathing.

When the muscle around the Dan Tien can be easily controlled, the process of breathing acts as a pump to start a fire, or Chi production, in the Dan Tien. In this respect, if deep breathing is the pump, then the Dan Tien is the furnace which must be activated in order to energize the Chi. By regular expansion of the Dan Tien, Chi begins to be generated and gathered in that area. This whole process of generating and accumulating Chi is called *lower level breathing,* while simple exhalation and inhalation in the lungs is called *upper level breathing.* One system aims at building Chi as energy, while the other aims at building up Chi as breath. The overabundant Chi in the Dan Tien will cause the abdominal area in most people to twitch and become warm. The pump, the deep breathing, has thus caused a fire, an accumulation of Chi, in the Dan Tien. When this occurs, the Chi is ready to burst out of the Dan Tien and travel into another cavity.

In order to insure that the accumulated Chi passes into the right cavity, the sitting posture must be correct (legs crossed). When the Chi is ready to burst from the Dan Tien, it must not be allowed to travel into the legs. By having the legs properly crossed, the Chi is effectively blocked from traveling into the legs via the meridians that pass into the lower extremities. If the Chi does pass into the legs, it can paralyze them. As a result, during any serious meditation session in which the practitioner attempts to circulate his Chi, the legs must be crossed. Only after the Small Circulation has been totally achieved and the meditator is attempting the Grand Circulation is it permissible to uncross the legs.

The next correct major cavity which the Chi must pass through to initiate Small Circulation is one located on the tailbone called Wei Lu. Thus the Chi passes down through the groin area, called the Bottom of the Sea in Chinese (Hai Di) and into the tailbone. The Chi does pass through other cavities on the way to the Wei Lu, but the Wei La will offer the greatest resistance. Therefore, it is imperative that the Chi pass easily through this first important obstacle. If the Chi gets stuck in this cavity, it could hurt the back and legs.

At this junction an extremely important point must be made. During meditation the mind must guide the Chi consciously throughout its circulation. Without the mind consciously leading the circulation of Chi, there will be no consistent or smooth circulation. It sometimes happens that the Chi will pass from the Dan Tien into the Wei Lu without conscious effort, but afterwards the mind must actively guide the Chi for further results. Starting from the Dan Tien, the mind remains calm and thoughtless about external worries while concentrating on guiding the Chi past the Wei Lu. This process must never be pushed. (The concentrated mind is one of the reasons why simple relaxation will only promote local circulation; for the larger circuits of circulation, Chi must be guided by the will.)

After the Chi has been successfully guided past the Wei Lu, it moves up the spine to the next major obstacle, the Jar Gi. The Jar Gi is located on the back directly behind the heart. Because this cavity is in a vital position, near the heart, the Chi must not get trapped; otherwise, the heart will be damaged.

Once the Chi passes the Jar Gi, the last major obstacle on the spine is the Yu Gen, the Jade Pillow, the cavity at the base of the skull. If the Chi is not passed smoothly through this point, it can pass into the nerves on the head, causing possible injury. The Yu Gen is called the Jade Pillow because that part of the head usually rests on the sleeping cushion. The above three major cavities are called Three Gates (Shan Gunn), in Chinese meditation.

After the Chi passes through the Yu Gen, the mind guides the Chi up over the head (Crown of the Head) (Tien Lien Gai), down the middle of the face and chest, and finally back to the Dan Tien, where the cycle will start over. When the complete cycle for Small Circulation has been achieved the whole process can be repeated again. When the practitioner has developed an easy flow of Chi in the pathway of the Small Circulation, the attempt to obtain the Grand Circulation may be tried. Usually, achieving Small Circulation requires three sessions of meditation per day for a period of ninety days. The Grand Circulation may take years to achieve.

Up to this point little has been said about the breathing act during Chi circulation. Now, with the basic background which the reader possesses, it is important to realize that in attempting to consciously pass the Chi through the various cavities on the path of the Small Circulation, and even after Small Circulation has been achieved, the cyclic movement of Chi must be exactly coordinated with the deep breathing process. Figure 1 shows the basic pattern which consists of guiding the Chi through one cycle of the Small Circulation by two sets of breaths. (Table 1 lists all the names of the important points and their corresponding abbreviations on Figures 1, 2, and 3.) This is the cycle that should be attempted by the beginner. To start, during the first inhalation the mind guides the Chi from the nose to the Dan Tien. Next, the practitioner exhales and guides the Chi from the Dan Tien to the Wei Lu. Then, he inhales and leads the Chi up to the point below the base of the neck called the Shun Bei. Finally, the practitioner exhales and guides the Chi over the head to the nose to complete one cycle. After completing one cycle, the same process is repeated.

After the two-breath cycle has been achieved, the Tai Chi practitioner should go on to circulating his Chi in an one-breath cycle. The one-breath cycle is the basis for using Chi as the energy source during Tai Chi fighting. Figure 2 shows the one-breath cycle. The practitioner guides the Chi to the tailbone while exhaling, and then to the nose while inhaling.

For the advanced practitioner, the current of Chi in the Small Circulation may be reversed so that the Chi travels up the chest, over the head, down the back, and then to the Dan Tien. In reverse circulation, the stopping points of Chi between inhalation and exhalation remain the same. Thus, inhale and guide the Chi from the Dan Tien to the nose; next, exhale and guide the Chi over the head to the Shun Bei. The next step is to inhale and guide the Chi to the tailbone or Wei Lu. Finally, exhale and guide the Chi to the Dan Tien. The one-breath cycle should follow the same principle.

Included with the one-breath cycle previously mentioned is the Buddhist system of Chi circulation: Figure 3. The Buddhist practitioner will inhale and guide his Chi from the nose, down the chest through the groin and to the tailbone. When he exhales, the Chi is guided up the spine, over the head, and to the

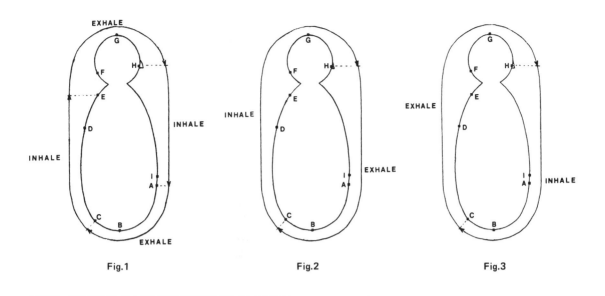

Fig.1   Fig.2   Fig.3

Table 1

Point	Name	Location	Cavity
A	Dan Tien	2" below navel	Yes
B	Hai Di	groin area	Yes
C	Wei Lu	tailbone	Yes
D	Jar Gi	behind heart on spine	Yes
E	Shun Bei	upper back	No
F	Yu Gen	base of skull	Yes
G	Tien Lien Gai	crown of head	Yes
H	Bi	nose	No
I	Du Gi	navel	No

nose. Buddhists can also reverse the direction of this cycle. The student should remember that in the Buddhist method the Dan Tien expands during inhalation and withdraws during exhalation.

Once the practitioner can pass this Chi through the Small Circulation, he may attempt Grand Circulation. For the achievement of Grand Circulation, the individual should stand as in Figure 4. In this standing position, the person can practice circulating his Chi into his arms or legs. To circulate Chi in the upper extremities, the individual's mind should guide the Chi in a complete circle through the curved arms. For the legs, only the leg that is on its toes should be practiced.

When the Tai Chi practitioner achieves a smooth flow of Chi through the Small Circulation he will only have begun to start the long road to martial proficiency. It will take years before the adept learns how to use the Chi from the Small Circulation for self-defense. But by devotion and diligent practice, the Tai Chi martial artist can make his system a beautiful yet deadly form of self-defense.

The Mechanics of Meditation

Points of Caution:

There are some general rules which the student should watch prior to and during meditation. Listed below are some of the important points:

1. Don't smoke. Because meditation involves deep breathing, the lungs will not function adequately.
2. Don't overuse alcohol. Too much alcohol will hurt the nervous system, thus hindering Chi circulation.
3. Clean the body before meditation. A clean body will relax the mind.
4. Wear comfortable clothing. Clothes, especially around the waist, should be loose. Tight clothes around the waist will make breathing difficult.
5. Meditate in a well-ventilated area. The air which one breathes should be as clean as possible.
6. Don't meditate 24 hours before or after sex.
7. Meditate in a quiet place with little or no disturbances.

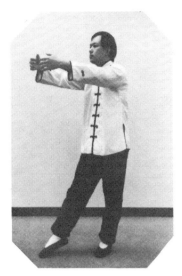
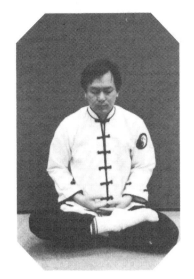
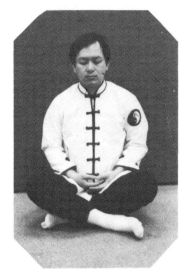

| Fig.4 | Fig.5 | Fig.6 |

Novice Meditators

The person who comes to meditation seriously for the first time should not attempt to circulate his Chi from the very start. The primary goal of the beginner must be to train the muscles around the Dan Tien so that the Taoist method of breathing is easy and natural. The training of the muscles is achieved through the preliminary practice of reverse breathing. Once the muscles have been adequately trained and the mind sufficiently calmed, the novice may then attempt to circulate his Chi.

Pre-meditation Warm-Up

Before meditation, the practitioner should spend 3 to 5 minutes calming down his mind. Once the mind is calm, one can begin concentrated meditation with better results. Calming the mind before meditation may be thought of as a warm-up exercise. For the more experienced person, the warm-up will take a shorter amount of time.

Posture

Basically, there are three cross-legged sitting positions which the meditator can assume: Figures 5, 6, and 7. The individual should pick the one that is most comfortable. In taking up any of these positions the back must remain as straight as possible but not stiff; do not slouch. Additionally, the individual should meditate on some sort of thick rug or pillow to help keep the back straight and balanced.

If while sitting the beginner's legs become numb, then he should uncross them and relax. Each time the novice should try to extend the time he remains seated so that the legs can bear up under the strain. In a few months the legs will feel no discomfort. To help relieve the cramping of the legs, the student can sit on the edge of a two inch mat. The student sits on the mat while the legs are in contact with the ground; the raised torso helps stop the legs from hurting excessively.

In all three sitting positions the hands are usually held at the Dan Tien (two inches below the navel) in an overlapping position. This positioning of the hands is normal for practitioners of Tai Chi during still meditation because it helps them feel their breathing as they attempt to expand the Dan Tien. This assists in coordinating deep breathing and Chi circulation. After the person has achieved Small Circulation, he may put the hands on the knees and lightly touch the thumb and middle finger.

Geographical Positioning

One should face the East while meditating or performing the Tai Chi sequences. This common practice was probably established because experienced meditators discovered that their Chi circulation was more fluid when facing the East. More efficient Chi circulation may come about when one faces East because the rotation of the earth geophysically helps the flow of Chi.

Position of Tongue, Teeth, and Eyes

During meditation the tongue should lightly press the roof of the mouth near the roof's center. By touching the tongue to the upper mouth cavity, a bridge is made between Yin and Yang. This bridge allows the Chi to circulate on a continuous path. The practitioner should watch that his tongue neither slips too far forward to too far back—both will hinder meditation. Additionally, the teeth should slightly touch. After meditation the teeth can be exercised by biting them together with moderate power. When the biting action occurs, the roots of the teeth are stimulated or exercised. This is one reason why people who eat meat often have strong teeth.

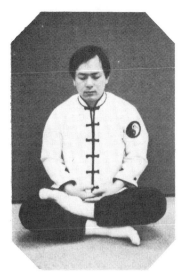
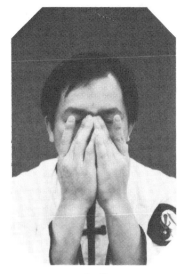
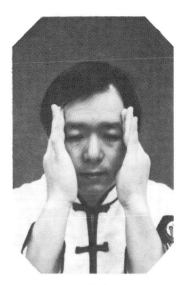

Fig.7   Fig.8   Fig.9

Besides building a bridge between the Yin and Yang, the upright tongue allows saliva to accumulate. The saliva should be periodically swallowed to lubricate the throat; otherwise, the throat will get too dry during meditation.

The eyes may be closed during meditation to help concentration. Although the eyes may be closed, the meditator should not let this make him sleepy. In such cases, the eyes may be half opened.

Time of Meditation

Usually, a person may meditate three times a day for sessions of one-half hour. If the individual decides to meditate three times a day, the best times to practice are 15 minutes before sunrise, 1 to 2 hours after lunch, and one-half hour before sleep. With this schedule, the meditator may, if his mind remains calm and concentrated, achieve Small Circulation in about three months.

The three times that are chosen for meditation have been found to be helpful for several reasons. By meditating before sunrise and in the evening, the individual will take advantage of the fact that the energy of his body changes from Yin to Yang. The other time is chosen because the individual is usually in a relaxed state during that period.

If a person can only meditate twice during the day, then the afternoon session should be skipped. If the meditator can only sit once during the day, then that one time can be in the morning or evening. With a reduced number of sessions, achieving Small Circulation will take a longer period of time.

Thoughts

During the meditation, the mind should focus on breathing and on the circulation of Chi. The whole purpose of meditation is lost if the mind wanders. The practitioner must, in a way, hypnotize himself into a relaxed state. One can easily achieve this relaxed state by concentrating on the rhymthmic pattern of breathing.

If the individual has too many day-to-day worries bothering him during meditation, then he should not attempt to meditate any futher nor attempt to circulate his Chi. Instead, the person can breathe deeply for relaxation. Attempting to circulate Chi during agitated mental states can only harm the meditator.

Role of the Instructor During Meditation

Oftentimes a Tai Chi instructor will meditate with his students. This is done for several reasons. First, if any trouble appears, the instructor is there to help the student. Second, after meditation the instructor can massage those people who need it. Third, by having an experienced instructor around during meditation, the instructor will implicitly create a suitable environment to circulate Chi.

Massage

After meditation, the student should always give himself a massage to readjust or redistribute the Chi around various areas of the body and to stimulate the main nerve systems. During meditation Chi will accumulate in some areas, therefore, the Chi needs to be spread around more evenly. Listed below are some important areas that need to be massaged.

Head: Begin with the face. Rub the eye bridge as in Figure 8, moving the hands up and across the forehead until the fingers pass the temple (Figure 9). Repeat several times. Next, put the hands under the eyes (Figure 10), and push them across the face sideways. Third, put the thumbs in

19

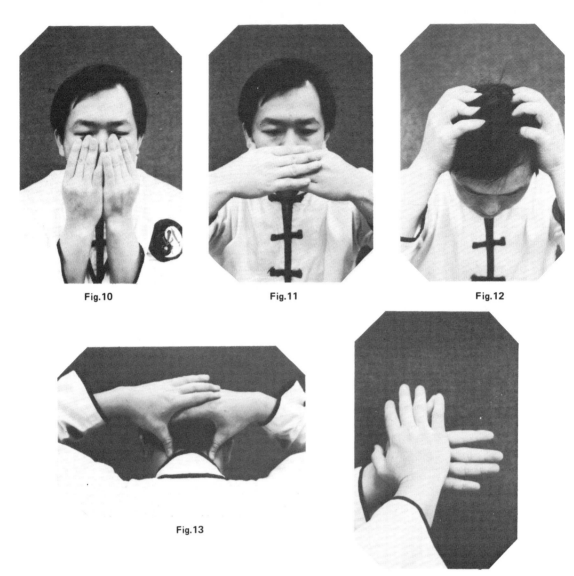

Fig.10　　　　　　　Fig.11　　　　　　　Fig.12

Fig.13

Fig.14

front of the ears (Figure 11), then move them down to the chin.

For the top of the head, place the fingers one inch off the centerline of the skull (Figure 12). Keep the fingers in place and gently rub the scalp. Reset the fingers along the same line, but toward the back, and gently rub again. Keep moving the fingers back along the head and massaging until the back of the skull is reached. One may also gently tap the head along the same line. This method of lightly tapping the head is called Min Gu or Beating the Drum. By gently tapping the head, the nerves are given a healthly stimulus, causing them to relax the muscle in the head.

The last place to rub in the head area is the neck. Place the thumbs at the base of the skull and push down (Figure 13).

Hands: Rub the palms together (Figure 14), then rub the center of the palm with the thumb (Figure 15). In the center of the palm is a cavity which lies on the kidney meridian. By massaging this cavity, the kidney is gently stimulated.

Kidneys: Form fists with both hands and place them on the back, behind the kidneys. Set the fists in one spot and rub with a circular motion (Figure 16).

Knees: During the meditation the knees may become stiff and absorb cold air through the pores. To warm up the knees and rid them of the cold air and stiffness, use the open hand to rub around the whole joint (Figure 17).

Foot: Take off your shoes and rub the center of the bottom of the foot (Figure 18). In this area lies a cavity which is part of the heart meridian.

20

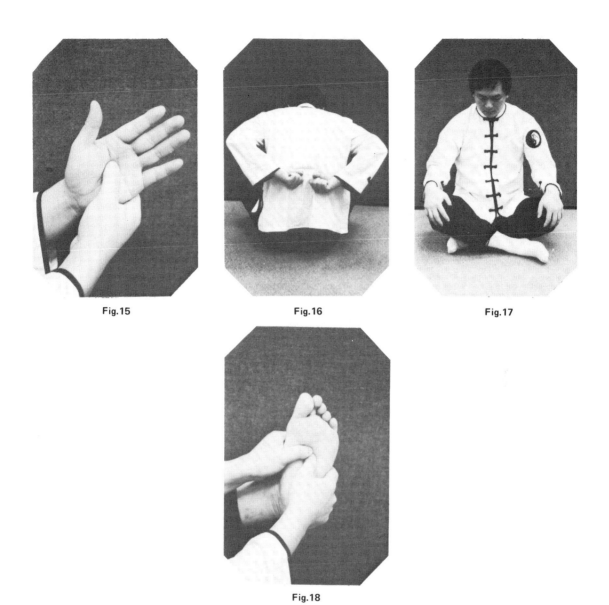

Fig. 15   Fig. 16   Fig. 17

Fig. 18

Internal Sounds: There are six sounds which a person can make which will relieve or stimulate certain internal organs in the individual. The basis for this practice can be easily seen in a person who is very sick. Very often the stricken individual will moan or sigh—these sounds are the same for all people around the world, whether in China, South America, or Australia, sick people make the same sounds. Basically, the function of these sounds is to relieve the inside organs of distress through the lungs. The six sounds which will be mentioned operate on the same principle.

These six sounds were originally taken from Buddhist medical sources. The sounds are Hur. Fu, Shyh, Shi, Shiu, and Chuei; they correspond to the heart, spleen, lung, triple burner, liver, and kidney. When each sound is made, dirty residual air is forced out. Because the dirty air occupies places that affect each organ, the organs themselves will benefit from the removal of the air. All the sounds must be sequentially done in one soft continuous breath—the sounds may be barely audible as they flow into one another.

Martial Applications of Tai Chi
Tai Chi Fighting Concepts

As a martial art, Tai Chi Chuan has evolved theories and practices which have come from hundreds of years of experience. These theories have developed in such a way that they are essentially geared to unite internal power with martial technique. Without martial technique, internal power is misdirected energy; without internal power, martial technique is a useless form. The unity of these two elements may be thought of as the key to Tai Chi fighting.

Before a person can correctly apply Tai Chi to actual fighting, two essential requirements are needed. First, the Tai Chi martial artist must have Grand Circulation to all parts of his body. The Chi must flow smoothly to any part of the body when the mind commands it. Second, the martial artist must coordinate the Grand Circulation with specific martial techniques. The second requirement develops out of intensive pushing hands practice. In all, fulfilling both requirements will take roughly two hours of practice every day for a period of ten years.

The first prerequisite of instantaneous Chi circulation to all parts of the body is mainly achieved by still meditation and by performing the Tai Chi sequences. Still meditation develops the Small Circulation while the moving sequence develops the Grand Circulation. Thus, for the Tai Chi martial artist, performing the slow motion sequence is of vital importance. Without using the slow sequence to circulate Chi smoothly, efficiently, and instantaneously, the martial artist cannot hope to generate the necessary internal power. As a result, the slow Tai Chi sequence is done at least three times during the day.

Once the slow motion barehand sequence can be done competently, the individual does the same sequence, but using speed and power to develop the martial applications of the techniques. Although the sequence is done with speed and power, the student must always keep his muscles relaxed; otherwise, only external not internal power will be built up. Basically, when the Tai Chi sequence is done with speed and power, there are three goals that must be achieved and eight general principles which must be observed for proficient use of martial technique. The first major goal is to gain stability by sinking the body. During any fast and powerful motion, the body must be balanced by having a firm foundation; without stability no base can exist for the actualization of power and technique. To produce a stable base in Tai Chi, the mind must mentally push the rear leg down and back, the striking arm must be mentally and physically pushed forward, and the Chi must be sunk straight down while expanding the Dan Tien. To perform all three actions in a coordinated action is to sink the body. When these three forces are balanced, the martial artist is in equilibrium, creating a foundation for the use of internal power and practical technique.

The second goal in performing the Tai Chi sequence with speed and power is to develop the ability to project power outwards in a short interval. The body must be relaxed and the muscles loose. While performing the fast sequence, the martial artist attempts to get his power out at the moment of the strike. Thus, the student must gain the capacity to send his Chi into the arm quickly and in a concentrated fashion so that it can be used for self-defense. Power, to be useful, must be instantaneous and concentrated.

To help the generation of instantaneous or quickly applied power, one must yell two sounds. Ha, the first sound, is used during the attacks. When ha is yelled out, the Dan Tien is made to expand and harden. This yelling assists the Chi into the arms. Hun, the second yell, is usually used during defense techniques such as dissolving and sticking; in this case, hun is made in the act of inhalation. Hun can also be used for attack with the act of exhalation. Besides helping the release of power, both yells are used to clear the lungs of dirty air and to distract an opponent.

The third goal of the fast Tai Chi sequence is the capacity to penetrate one's power beyond the surface level of attack. This goal requires that the practitioner develop the calmness of a mountain and the movements of a stream; the martial artist must be powerful and fluid at the same time. These traits are extremely hard to develop because any time that someone engages in fast motion, their nerves have a tendency to become overstimulated, causing the body to tighten. Secondly, to obtain suitable levels of penetration, the person must know the purpose of each technique. By knowing the practical application of every technique, the student will know the exact nature and amount of power which is required.

From years of experience, Tai Chi stylists have found that the penetration of power is more advantageously trained when a person practices the techniques against an imaginary opponent. By pretending to actually fight against an opponent, the martial artist develops the habit of using real and effective power. This will also help actual Chi circulation.

As previously mentioned, there are also eight principles which must be followed and which summarize all the major goals to be aimed at while performing fast Tai Chi. The first four major principles are extremely important for explaining the mechanics of a technique in action. To begin, the foot is the root of the body; the feet are the points from which stability emerges. Next, the legs are the power source in Tai Chi. While the Chi which is produced in the Dan Tien is the energy for martial power, as gasoline is energy for a car, the legs are the medium through which energy expresses itself. As an example, when a person pushes a heavy box, he can feel both legs exert pressure on the floor while pushing the box. If the same person attempted to push the heavy box while standing straight up, or in a position from which the legs cannot push, the box would be almost impossible to move because the power source is gone. As an extension of this, if the Tai Chi practitioner can circulate Chi into his legs, he will then give the legs an enormous energy source for pushing backwards; the greater the backward push of the legs, the greater the forward push of the arms. Third, the waist is the control or the rudder for the direction and application of power. It is the waist that guides the power generated in the legs. Last and fourth, the hands feel the opponent's power and then the fingers and palms express the power for real results.

The next four principles which direct the Tai Chi martial artist during training are the possession of a light body, smooth Chi circulation, fullness of Chi, and a calm spirit. These four ideas complement and realize the first principles. Together, all eight must be strictly observed.

In addition to the elements previously discussed, a few more general remarks may be stated about Tai Chi free fighting. Whenever a Tai Chi stylist fights, one of his major aims is to use, direct, and reflect the opponent's power against himself. For this reason, Tai Chi specializes in short and middle range fighting. (Roughly, the short range is when two people stand at arms' length, and middle range is when two people stand slightly beyond arms' length.)

Because the Tai Chi student wants to use his opponent's power, he will usually fight defensively instead of offensively. Many times while fighting in the short and middle range, the Tai Chi practitioner will push his opponent down to stop aggression in a relatively peaceful manner. By pushing an opponent down, one warns the other side that he could have made the push into a full strike.

Another characteristic of the Tai Chi styles is the tendency to strike only particular areas. These areas are usually the chest, back, side of the neck, back of the head, the knee, and the groin. Generally, by striking those areas, an opponent can be disabled while avoiding the necessity of a death blow. In particular, Tai Chi practitioners specialize in a technique called *sealing the breath or vein.* In this special technique, the chest, back, or side of the neck are stuck in certain zones with the palm or forearm. When those zones are attacked, they will either prevent the lungs from taking oxygen or the veins and arteries in the neck from transporting blood to the brain. The end result of sealing the breath or vein is unconsciousness since either attack will cause insufficient oxygen in the brain. This technique requires the use of internal power.

In terms of actual forms, the thirteen postures have evolved into a set of techniques which are characteristic of Tai Chi. The thirteen postures represent, in total, the various directions and methods of movement. But for the various directions, N, E, W, S, NE, NW, SW, and SE, Tai Chi stylists have assigned eight techniques which can neutralize attacks from each specific direction. The techniques can be interchanged, but traditionally they have been assigned to certain directions.

Tai Chi Power

The major difference between Tai Chi Chuan and other martial styles is in the development and use of power. In Tai Chi the major emphasis is on methods that build up and refine various types of internal power for assorted situations. Tai Chi, more than other styles, has refined the types and kinds of power to an exacting degree. In this section, the characteristics of Tai Chi power will be delineated so that the reader will have a general idea of its nature.

To understand Tai Chi power, it would be convenient to compare it to external power. In comparing both types of power, Tai Chi power can be seen to have six major characteristics. First, Tai Chi uses circular power in resolving, dissolving, and neutralizing attacks. Tai Chi's defensive power guides rather than stops an opponent's attack. In contrast, external power is square. When a person using external power is put on the defensive, he must more or less stop an attack by a violent linear block.

Second, Tai Chi power is shapeless or formless. When a Tai Chi martial artist uses his power, his muscles don't tense up or become violently agitated. Instead, when a Tai Chi practitioner uses his power the muscles are relaxed and smooth. However, one can see the shape of external power—the muscles tense in preparation for violent motion.

The third distinguishing trait of Tai Chi power is its speed. Speed in this context means that more power is delivered in a shorter time period. External power, however, delivers its impact over a wider interval of time than internal power. Tai Chi power is more like an explosion, while external power is like an extended push. If a person is struck by an accomplished Tai Chi martial artist, the victim will seem to fly back as if suddenly hit by a fast moving truck.

Fourth, Tai Chi power is more focused and concentrated than external power. In Tai Chi, more power can be delivered into a given area. External power is more diluted or diffuse than Tai Chi power.

The fifth characteristic of Tai Chi power is its sunkeness and stability. When a technique is performed with power, the student has his legs firmly rooted to the ground while the joints hang down in a sunken position. As a result, Tai Chi commonly contains no jumping kicks or punches which require that the body leave the ground. On the other hand, external power floats higher in the body in an excited state. The styles that use external power generate it mainly from the waist and shoulders.

Last, Tai Chi power has an acute ability to penetrate beyond the surface of attack. The power which a Tai Chi martial artist generates can go deep into an opponent's body in a focused manner. For this reason Tai Chi martial artists also specialize in a technique called *cavity press*. In cavity press the practitioner penetrates his power into acupuncture points to pass the destructive power into the meridian. From the meridian, the power goes into a particular internal organ. In addition, the stylist may also send his power directly into an internal organ causing it to literally explode. Such strikes produce no external bruises because the power went beyond the surface skin and muscle. External power, in comparison, is usually duller, stopping at or a little beneath the surface. Some people who use external power can, through years of practice, achieve a good deal of penetration, but it will not be as much as if the power was internal.

The six characteristics of Tai Chi power only describe it in general terms, but to be more specific requires the use of key words. Key words are a list of traits, tendencies, habits, strategies, techniques, etc., that form the basis for the martial theories of a specific style. The key words may be said to define the unique personality of a martial style. In Yang's style of Tai Chi there are twenty-five key words which describe the foundation of the system. Of the twenty-five key words, seventeen are related to the application and type of power. The remaining eight describe the original techniques mentioned in the previous section. Listed below are the key words of Tai Chi:

key words of Tai Chi

1. Adhere or stick	2. Listening	3. Understanding
4. Retreat	5. Neutralize	6. Ward-Off
7. Roll Back	8. Press	9. Push
10. Rend	11. Shoulder-stroke	12. Elbow-stroke
13. Pluck	14. Guide	15. Grasp
16. Release	17. Borrow	18. Open
19. Close	20. Raise	21. Sink
22. Extend	23. Intercept	24. Screw
25. Jump		

In this section only the first five will be described. The eight techniques (6-13) may be found in the barehand and fighting sequence. The remaining key words (14-25) can be researched by the reader as he studies and practices Tai Chi.

The first five key words are unique to Tai Chi. These five words contain the most fundamental aspects of Tai Chi as a martial art. When an individual has mastered the meaning and ability of each key word, then that person can be truly described as a true stylist.

To begin, when a Tai Chi martial artist engages in combat, his first action is to Adhere or Stick to his opponent. By adhering, the defender prevents his enemy from escaping and launching a new attack. If the person adheres properly, he will follow the attacker's power very easily. This type of power sucks in and clings to the enemy, thus beginning the process of counterattack.

A famous story exists about Yang Chien Huo which demonstrates the unique ability of sinking and adhering. To test Yang Chien Huo's capacity of adhering and neutralizing power, a bird was placed on his open palm. When the bird attempted to fly away it could not. Everytime the bird started to push off Yang Chien Huo's hand to initiate flight, the great master followed the bird's power, giving the creature no base from which to start flight. The ability to adhere comes from the constant and concentrated practice of pushing hands.

Once the practitioner sticks onto his opponent, the defender will listen to the enemy's power. The Tai Chi martial artist will not listen with his ears, but with his developed sense of touch. Through years of practice, the defender's skin can feel the slightest movement of the opponent. By possessing the ability to listen to an attacker's movements, any action can be anticipated. Listening is gained through practicing pushing hands.

Because the act of listening is passive knowledge, the Tai Chi martial artist must then understand or actively interpret his opponent's action and power. In understanding an attacker's movements, Tai Chi practitioners have set up four basic guidelines for understanding: first, if the enemy moves fast, the defender moves fast; second, if the enemy moves slow, the defender moves slow; third, if the enemy does not move, the defender does not move; and fourth, if the enemy moves slightly, the defender moves first.

After the opponent's actions are understood, then the defender retreats to avoid the enemy's power in order that neutralization or counterattack may be started. Usually, adhering plus retreating will equal the neutralization. If each step is done quickly and with expertise, the process will end with the defeat of the opponent. Such skill only will come about through years of practice.

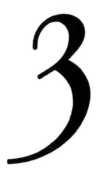

BAREHAND TAI CHI CHUAN

To competently execute the barehand techniques of Tai Chi, this chapter will present and explain fundamental methods of training, the Tai Chi barehand sequence, pushing hands and the Tai Chi fighting sequence. Taken together, these elements will lay a foundation for the reader in self-defense and health. By paying careful attention to the instructions and by diligent practice, the reader may easily catch the major principles and forms so that each technique can be done with relative smoothness.

Fundamental Practice

In this section, the foundation for the barehand techniques will be shown, including hand forms, stances, and fundamental drills, both stable and moving. The hand forms and stances will be essentially geared so that the student will have correct forms, while the fundamental drills basically serve another purpose. The fundamental drills were constructed so that they could be easily coordinated with the inhalation and exhalation of deep breathing. While the easily performed fundamental drills include martial techniques, they help the beginner develop Taoist breathing because they are simple in form; the novice can practice deep breathing instead of concentrating his mind on remembering the correct outer form. The fundamental drills are also used as warm-up exercises to calm the mind and regulate the breath before actual performance of the Tai Chi sequence.

As a final note, the last two stable fundamental breathing drills, Gung-Lu (Surround and Rollback) and An (Press), are the most important of this whole group. Both are very important for developing Chi circulation and correct charge distribution in the arms. These two drills are also useful in obtaining relaxation and concentration.

Hand Forms

In Tai Chi there are basically two hand forms: the open palm and the fist (Figures 1 and 2). While practicing the fundamental drills or while doing the Tai Chi sequence, both forms are relaxed and loose. The wrist should never be made tight. When using the open palm, the thumb should be set back slightly, as if the hand were cupping a spherical object, but not allowing the thumb to touch the round object.

Stances

Tai Chi, like other martial arts has its own fundamental stances that are the basis for stability, movement, and martial technique. Basically, Tai Chi uses eight stances (Ba Shih), each of which is used during the barehand sequence. Described below are the eight stances. The reader can ignore the positioning of the hands until he begins the sequence.

Ma Bu (Figure 3)

Ma Bu, or the Horse Stance, is commonly used as a transition between techniques and forms. To assume this stance, first place the feet parallel, slightly beyond shoulder width. Next, turn and bend the knees in slightly. Both feet must remain flat.

Deng San Bu (Figure 4)

This important form, the Mountain Climbing Stance, is the most commonly used offensive stance in Tai Chi. First, place one leg forward so that the knee is above the ankle, and the leg as a whole supports 60 percent of the body's weight. The toe of the lead leg is pointing 15 degrees to the inside. The rear leg is firmly set down while supporting the rest of the weight. The knee of the rear leg must be slightly bent in this stance. Keep the upper body perpendicular to the ground.

Dsao Pan Bu (Figure 5)

Dsao Pan Bu, the Sitting on Crossed Legs Stance, is the most commonly used stance for forward

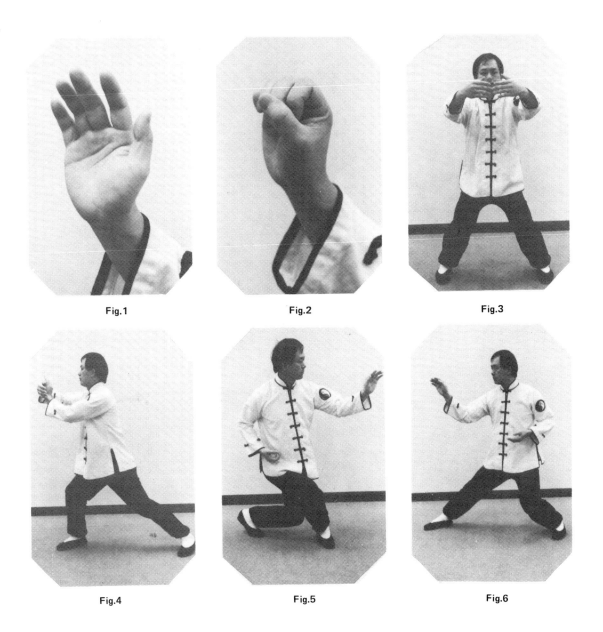

Fig.1   Fig.2   Fig.3

Fig.4   Fig.5   Fig.6

movement. First, assume Ma Bu. Second, turn the body and the right foot 90 degrees clockwise while pivoting on the left toe. The same can be done with the left side: turn the body and the left foot 90 degrees counterclockwise, and pivot on the right foot. From either side, the rear leg can easily move forward.

Ssu Lieu Bu (Figure 6)

This form, the Four-Six Stance, is the most commonly used defensive stance in Tai Chi. In weight distribution, it is exactly the opposite of Deng San Bu; the front leg supports 40 percent of the weight and the rear leg 60 percent. The rear leg is turned inward with the front leg flexible, bent, and relaxed.

Fu Hu Bu (Figure 7)

Fu Hu Bu, or Tame the Tiger Stance, is used for low attacks and defense. To assume Fu Hu Bu, stand with both feet spread. Next, squat down on one leg while keeping the other leg locked. The thigh of the squatting leg must be parallel to the ground and both feet must lie flat.

Shuen Gi Bu (Figure 8)

Shuen Gi Bu, called the False Stance, is used to set up kicks. First, place all your weight on one leg. Next, set the other leg in front of the body with only its toes lightly touching the ground. From this position the false leg can kick without hesitation.

27

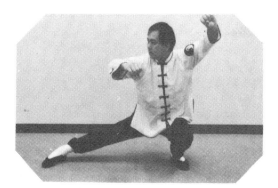

Fig.7

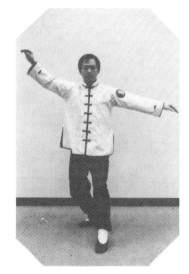

Fig.8

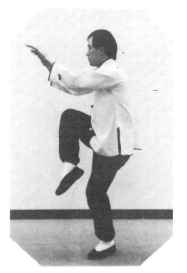

Fig.9

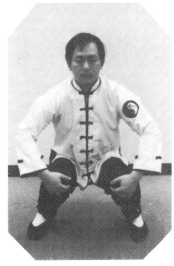

Fig.10

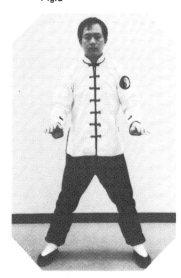

Fig.11

Gin Gi Du Li (Figure 9)

Gin Gi Du Li, the Golden Rooster Standing on One Leg Stance, is similar in form to Shuen Gi Bu and serves the same function; to set up kicks. To assume this stance lift either knee up with the toe pointing 45 degrees down. The raised leg can kick at any instant.

Dsao Dun (Figure 10)

Dsao Dun, the Squat Stance, is primarily used as a training device to build up the knees. To begin, stand with feet spread shoulder width apart. Squat down until the thighs are parallel to the ground and the back is straight. The reader should attempt to stay in this stance for five minutes while keeping the mind calm.

Fundamental Drills: Stable

The first fundamental drill which the beginner should practice is Tou Tien or Supporting the Heaven. This training method was constructed to develop endurance while strengthening the knees. Because Tai Chi martial artists generate power from their legs, this form is extremely important. While performing Tou Tien, the practitioner should breathe deeply and keep his mind off pain and stress. In Tai Chi, the training methods develop both mind and body.

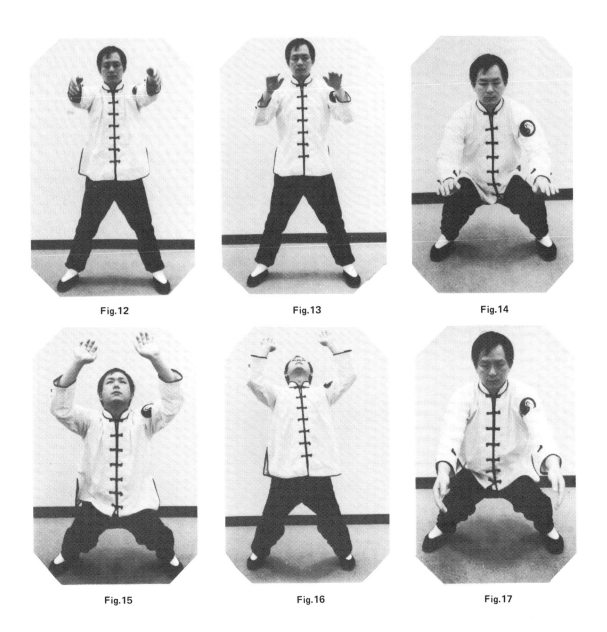

Fig.12　　　　　　　　Fig.13　　　　　　　　Fig.14

Fig.15　　　　　　　　Fig.16　　　　　　　　Fig.17

To start Tou Tien, stand with the hands at the waist, palms down, in a relaxed position (Figure 11). Breathe deeply a few times to calm the mind. Raise the arms while turning the palms toward each other (Figure 12), and breathe in. Turn the palms face down (Figure 13), and squat down into Dsao Dun while exhaling (Figure 14). Remain in Dsao Dun and raise the arms above the head while inhaling (Figure 15). The forearms are then parallel pushing up, and the face looks up while exhaling. The practitioner should stay locked in the form shown in Figure 16 for at least five minutes; the stance is changed to Ma Bu.

Once the five minutes are up, lower the body down into Dsao Dun while keeping the arms above the head and inhaling. Lower the arms to the front of the body and exhale (Figure 17). Slowly raise the body into the position shown in Figure 12, inhaling at the same time. Finally, exhale and lower the arms down into their original position (Figure 11).

The next ten fundamental drills are all done from an upright position and involve little or no movement by the legs. Their basic purpose is to allow the individual to practice deep breathing in coordination with physical movement. If the person cannot practice the Tai Chi sequence for some reason, then he may perform the fundamental drills each morning to calm the mind and freshen the body. In executing each form, the body must be relaxed and the mind peaceful.

29

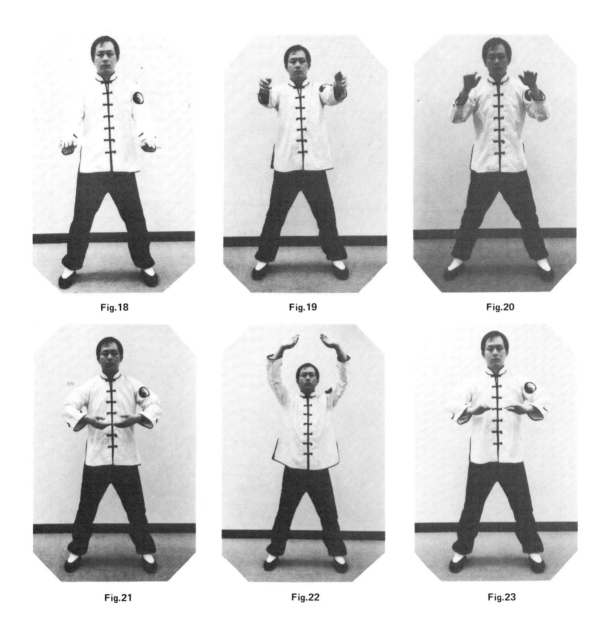

Fig.18   Fig.19   Fig.20

Fig.21   Fig.22   Fig.23

Fundamental Breathing Drill 1

Figure 18: Place the hands at the waist, palms down. Inhale and exhale.

Figure 19: Turn the palms in and raise the arms to shoulder height. Inhale.

Figure 20: Turn the palms down and return to the original position of Figure 18, while exhaling.

Fundamental Breathing Drill 2

Figure 21: Assume the position in Figure 18. Bring the hands to the center of the body, while turning the palms up. Inhale.

Figure 22: Move both arms up while turning the palms up, exhaling at the same time.

Figure 23: Turn the palms down, lower the arms, and return to the original position. Inhale and exhale.

Fundamental Breathing Drill 3

Figure 24: Assume the position in Figure 18. Raise and cross the arms so that the palms face in. Begin inhalation.

Figure 25: Raise both arms up, out and then down. Exhale when the arms are going down.

Fundamental Breathing Drill 4

Figure 26: Assume the position in Figure 18. Raise the arms up and out to the sides, palms facing up. Inhale. Continue to raise the arms above the head, then down across the body to the original position. Exhale. This form is the reverse of number 3.

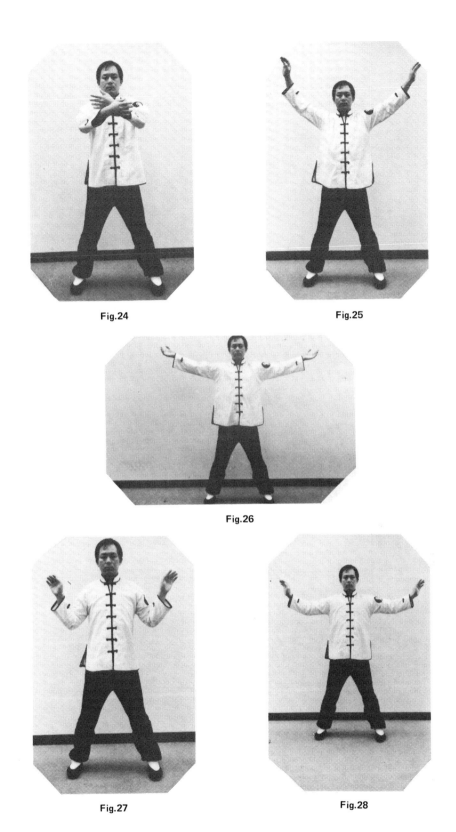

Fig.24

Fig.25

Fig.26

Fig.27

Fig.28

Fundamental Breathing Drill 5

Figure 27: Assume position in Figure 18. Raise the arms up as in Figure 21. When the arms reach shoulder height, turn the palms out. Inhale.

Figure 28: Push the arms to the side and exhale. Bring the arms back to the position in Figure 27 and inhale. To end the cycle, lower the arms to the original position and exhale.

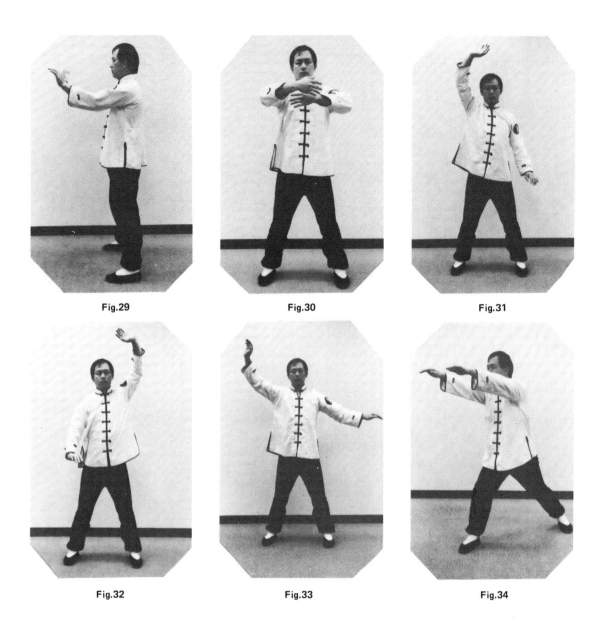

Fig.29   Fig.30   Fig.31

Fig.32   Fig.33   Fig.34

Fundamental Breathing Drill 6

Figure 29: Assume the position in Figure 18. Raise the arms as in Figure 21. Turn the palms forward when the arms reach shoulder height. Inhale. Next, push both arms forward and exhale. Bring the arms back. Inhale. Lower the arms to the original position and exhale.

Fundamental Breathing Drill 7

Figure 30: Assume the position in Figure 18. Raise both arms, palms facing in, to shoulder height. Inhale.

Figure 31: Raise the right arm, palm up, while lowering the left arm, palm down. Exhale.

Figure 32: Return both arms to the position in Figure 30. Inhale. Raise the left arm, palm up, while lowering the right arm, palm down. Exhale.

Fundamental Breathing Drill 8

Figure 33: Assume the position in Figure 18, and raise both arms as in Figure 30. Inahle. When the arms are at shoulder height, spread them out so the right arm is higher than the left. Exhale. Bring the arms back to the position in Figure 30. Inhale. Spread the arms again with the left hand higher than the right. Exhale.

Fundamental Breathing Drill 9 (Gung-Lu)

Figure 34: Assume Deng San Bu and extend both arms so they are parallel, palms facing down.

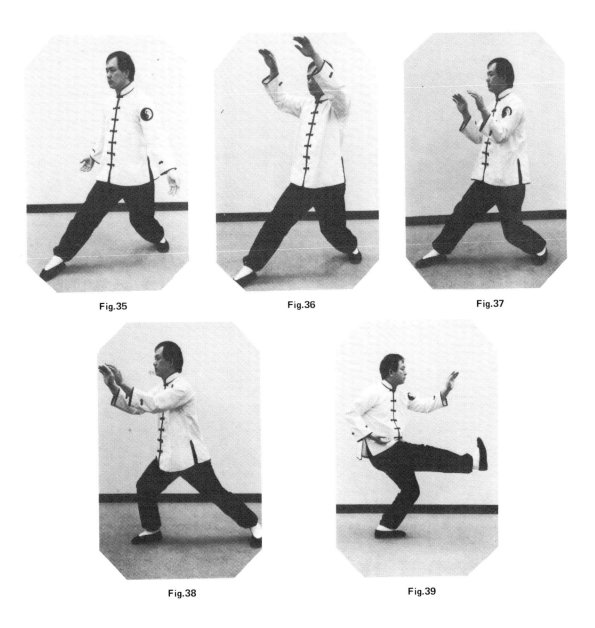

Fig.35   Fig.36   Fig.37

Fig.38   Fig.39

Figure 35: Shift the weight back so the stance is Ssu Lieu Bu while slowly moving the arms down past the forward knee, palms turned up. Next, raise both arms straight up until they are at shoulder height. Inhale. Shift the weight forward so the stance is Deng San Bu while swinging the arms forward horizontally, thus assuming the original position. Exhale. Repeat the cycle 20 times with the right leg forward, and 20 times with the left leg forward.

Fundamental Breathing Drill 10 (An)

Figure 36: Start in Ssu Lieu Bu and raise both arms up. Begin to inhale.

Figure 37: Bring both arms down to the front of the chest. Complete inhalation.

Figure 38: Shift the stance forward to Deng San Bu and push forward with both arms. Exhale. Repeat the cycle 20 times with the right leg forward and 20 times with the left leg forward.

Fundamental Moving Drills

Fundamental Moving Drill 1

Figure 39: To begin, stand with the feet shoulder width apart. Raise the right knee and inhale. Slowly kick the right leg out while moving the left hand forward. When the left hand is at the waist, its palm faces up. As the hand comes forward, the palm is turned out. Exhale. Set the right leg down and withdraw the left hand to the waist. Once the right leg is set, lift the left knee. Inhale. Slowly kick the left leg out while pushing the right hand forward. Exhale. Set the left leg down and repeat the cycle. This form is called Chai Twe and means the Step on Kick.

33

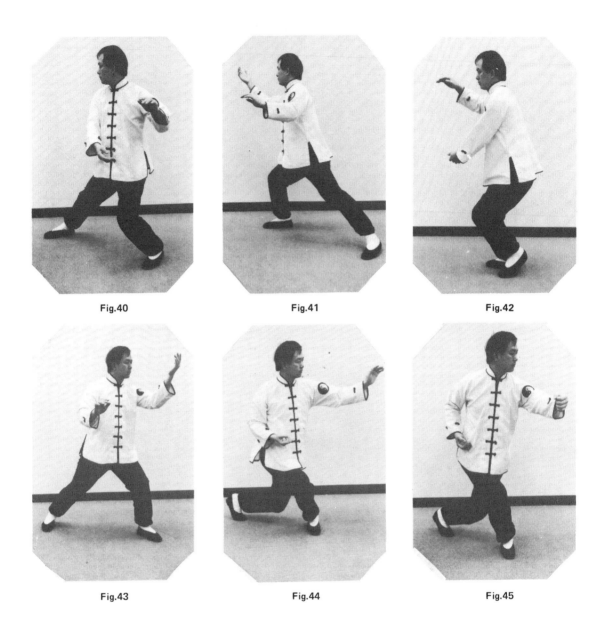

Fig.40   Fig.41   Fig.42

Fig.43   Fig.44   Fig.45

Fundamental Moving Drill 2

Figure 40: This drill is called Yeh Ma Fen Tsung or Wild Horses Share the Mane. Start by standing with the feet shoulder width apart. Move the right leg forward at a 45 degree angle, sliding the left arm up, palm down, and the right arm down, palm up. Inhale.

Figure 41: Shift the stance to Deng San Bu while sliding the right hand up. Exhale.

Figure 42: Bring the left leg forward and turn the right palm down and the left palm up. Inhale.

Figure 43: Step 45 degrees to the left while shifting the stance to Deng San Bu. Slide the left hand up. Exhale. Bring the right leg forward and turn the left palm down and the right palm up. Inhale. Step 45 degrees to the right and repeat the cycle.

Fundamental Moving Drill 3

Figure 44: This exercise is called Pieh Shen Chui or the Circle Punch. Assume Deng San Bu, right leg forward. Turn the right leg out and shift the stance to Dsao Pan Du (inhale) while circling the right fist in a clockwise motion in front of the body (exhale). As the hand completes the circle, it retreats to the waist, palm up, while the left hand swings to the front.

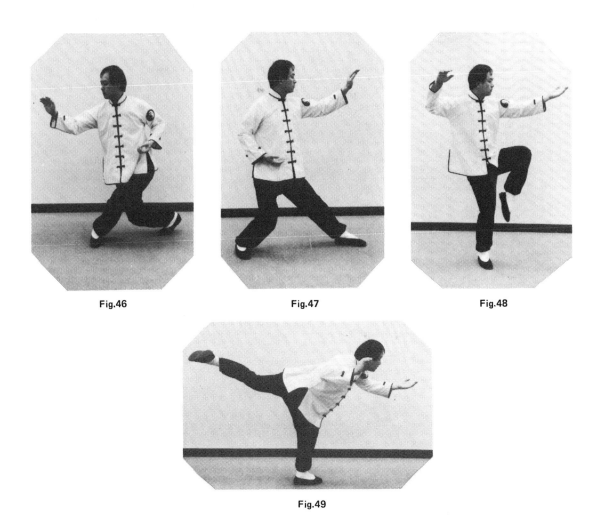

Fig.46   Fig.47   Fig.48

Fig.49

Figure 45: The left hand begins to make a counterclockwise circle, in a fist, to the front of the body. Inhale.

Figure 46: As the left hand makes the circle, step forward with the left leg into Dsao Pan Bu. Withdraw the left hand to the waist, palm up, while swinging the right hand across the body. Exhale. Circle the right fist in front of the body and repeat the cycle.

Fundamental Moving Drill 4

Figure 47: This drill is called Tao Nien Hou or Repulse the Monkey. Start with the left leg forward in Ssu Lieu Bu, left hand forward, palm out. Begin to inhale.

Figure 48: Circle the left hand counterclockwise until the palm faces up, while the right hand moves back and up. At the same time that the hands are moving, lift the left knee. Complete inhalation.

Figure 49: Turn on the right heel so that the right foot is pointing forwards. Exhale. Extend the left leg straight back while tilting the upper body forward for balance. The hands remain in the same position. Inhale. Step down with the left leg and push forward with the right hand, while retreating the left hand to the waist. The stance is Ssu Lieu Bu. Exhale when the left leg touches down. Repeat the entire process for the right side. Reverse all the directions for right and left. Keep the breathing the same.

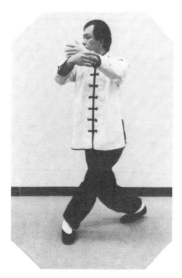 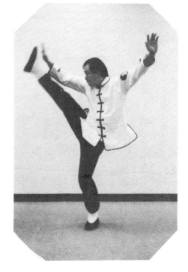

Fig.50   Fig.51

Fundamental Moving Drill 5

Figure 50: This drill is called Tso Yu Fen Chiao or the Left-Right Kick. Start with legs shoulder width apart. Step forward with the left leg into Dsao Pan Bu while crossing the arms to the side. Inhale.

Figure 51: Spread the arms open and snap kick with the right leg, slapping the right hand. Exhale. Cross the arms again, except off to the right side. Inhale. Spread the arms open and snap kick with the left leg, slapping the left hand. Exhale. Set the left leg down and repeat from the beginning. On all the kicks the base leg must remain flat.

Tai Chi Barehand Sequence

The barehand sequence which is presented in its entirety in this chapter is the traditional one practiced by the stylists of Yang's Tai Chi Chuan. In the traditional barehand sequence, the apparent number of techniques vary between 81 and 150, depending on the method used to count and group the forms. Some instructors and writers, for example, will not count repeated forms. But basically, the reader may judge whether a Tai Chi sequence is complete by comparing the arrangement of the names given to the techniques. While the methods of counting the techniques vary, the names and their arrangement do not.

If an instructor has taken out techniques to shorten the sequence, the practitioner should practice the sequence several times to receive the health benefits of Tai Chi. As was stated in the Preface, the original sequence was constructed to have enough forms to achieve results beneficial to health; shortening the sequence shortens the time of exercise.

When a person does the Tai Chi sequence, his ultimate aim is the achievement of a near mystic state. As the practitioner does the sequence, he should lose all feeling for his own personal existence. All the problems and worries of his life should disappear into nothingness. Eventually, the individual will experience his body spread wide into the universe while becoming transparent. At the same time, the Chi circulates easily and smoothly. When the individual reaches this condition, he is truly in a state of moving meditation.

If the practitioner is interested in developing the martial aspect of Tai Chi, he should do the entire sequence three continuous times each morning. But if the individual is only interested in the health aspect of Tai Chi, then the sequence can be performed once each morning.

During the morning itself, the best time to practice is before sunrise so that the person can take advantage of the change in the Yin and Yang energies of the body. Because the sequence should take at least 20 minutes to perform, it must be done 20 minutes before the sun comes up.

By doing the sequence in a minimum of 20 minutes, the inhalations and exhalations will be relatively equal. Therefore, the beginner should not let the sequence take less than this time. Later, as the individual becomes more proficient, he can extend the time. A time of 30 minutes for one sequence is very good. The ultimate goal is to perform one complete set in 60 minutes. To achieve a time of 60 minutes requires slow, but consistent breathing, and a highly concentrated, yet relaxed, mind: the practitioner is in a semiconscious state while the body moves slowly.

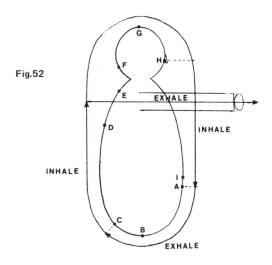

Fig.52

For the individual who practices Tai Chi for improved health and who does not meditate in order to circulate Chi, performing the Tai Chi sequence with the proper series of deep breaths while maintaining a relaxed body will have the desired results. In this state, the Chi will naturally circulate.

For the person practicing Tai Chi as a martial art, once he has achieved fluid Chi circulation during the barehand sequence, he should perform the sequence with speed and power. The fast sequence should be practiced at least once during the day. Without performing the barehand techniques with speed and power, the techniques cannot be made effective. For all the key points of combat Tai Chi, refer to Chapter 2.

In terms of the practical aspects of barehand Tai Chi, listed below are major areas which the student should be aware of.

Breathing

During each sequence the practitioner uses the Taoist method of deep breathing: withdraw the Dan Tien while inhaling, and expand the Dan Tien while exhaling. Every breath must be coordinated with the application of the techniques. Every time a defensive maneuver is performed, inhale; every time an offensive move is performed, exhale. Keep the tongue gently pressed against the roof of the mouth and breathe through the nose. Swallow all the saliva that is produced to keep the throat moist. If a particularly long Tai Chi form requires that the practitioner extend his breath beyond his natural capacity, he may add a series of shorter breaths to the technique.

Warm Up

Before practicing the sequence, the individual should stretch his legs out and then calm his mind by doing fundamental breathing drills. Because there are kicks in the sequence, the muscles must be properly loosened to avoid injury. To fully receive the benefits of the sequence, the mind must enter the performance in a tranquil state: otherwise, too much time will be spent during the sequence in calming the mind.

Chi Circulation During Barehand Tai Chi

In the section on meditation, the Chi cycle for Small Circulation was explained in detail for sitting meditation. But in the moving Tai Chi sequence, the path of the Chi through the Small Circulation is slightly different. The Chi cycle during barehand Tai Chi is shown in Figure 52. As the practitioner inhales, the Chi is brought from the tailbone up the back to the base of the neck. Inhaling also prepares the Chi on the front side of the body for a new cycle. When the practitioner exhales, the Chi is guided by the mind, not over the head, but into the arms. At the same time that the Chi flows into the arm, the Dan Tien expands, starting a new cycle by moving the new Chi into the tailbone. Once the practitioner inhales again, he guides the Chi to the base of the neck while preparing for a new cycle on the front of the body. Thus, the Chi cycle during moving meditation is a one way path, in that it does not travel in a complete circle, but in a line that ends in the hands.

Because the Chi is guided into the arm, Tai Chi stylists will feel their palms and arms tingle and become warm. These sensations are produced by the energy of Chi. Even individuals who have not passed fully, or not at all, through the Small Circulation have been able to feel these sensations in their arms and palms, in as little as six months. In these particular cases, the individuals have only developed the local circulation of Chi in their arms and palms. While the local circulation of Chi is good in terms of health, it is not enough for martial purposes.

Position and Posture of the Body

To obtain the greatest benefits from Tai Chi, the body should be in a proper posture during the bare-hand sequence. First, the fingers, wrist, arms, and shoulders, must be relaxed and held low, not high and tense. Always keep the elbows down; raising the elbows excessively causes poor martial form and tense muscles. Secondly, the spine and the whole upper body must be straight. When the body is straight, the front and back muscles are equally relaxed, making the Chi flow with the same ease on both sides. In addition, when the spine is straight, the internal organs are not packed over each other, hindering blood circulation. Finally, the sequence should be performed in a quiet and refreshing place while facing the East.

Movement

All the movements in the sequence are done lightly and without heavy steps. Each step is done as if the person were on ice: gently and softly. In the sequence there are many moves in which the practitioner must turn his body to an opposite direction without lifting the legs. In these particular instances, turning must be done on the heels, one at a time, in a smooth wave.

Power Generation

Besides using the slow motion sequence to help the circulation of Chi, the Tai Chi martial artist also uses it to build up the potential for power. To approach this goal, every time that the practitioner pushes or punches out, the Chi is sunk into the Dan Tien, the rear leg is mentally pushed back, and the power is applied in the hand. These three power vectors (forward, down, and back) are necessary to develop the kind of stable and symmetrical power used by Tai Chi stylists. Although the power is developed out of the three vectors, the muscles must never become tight. The martial power must be generated from the Chi, not the muscles.

Yelling

In the Tai Chi sequence there are a few places that contain fast motion and will require that the performer yell "Ha." The yell should come from deep in the lungs, not from the throat. While yelling, the Dan Tien must expand. The yell will clear out the dirty air in the lungs. The times at which to yell will be stated in the description of the sequence.

External Movements

There are six traits which the individual should keep in mind while performing barehand Tai Chi. These points are smoothness, balance, centering, relaxation, continuity, and coordination of mind, body, and breath. By noting these points while someone does the Tai Chi sequence, he can judge the performer's mastery of the forms.

Imagined Opponent

To help with total form, the practitioner should imagine that he is using each technique against an imaginary opponent. This will make each technique more accurate and help with the circulation of Chi. While also thinking about the make believe opponent, the performer must come to think of his waist as the first master, the throat as the second master because it controls the yell, and the heart as the third master because it guides the mind.

Direction For The Tai Chi Sequence

In the photographs of the sequence, only those that contain the lone individual in the white top are part of the regular solo sequence. Those photographs that contain two individuals show the specific applications of each technique. By showing the specific use of each form, the practitioner will have a better notion of the function and structure of the technique. Even though the Tai Chi sequence may be performed strictly for exercise, the forms should at least be accurate in martial terms. For the solo barehand pictures, the photographs represents the correct form. As a result, many details were left out in the written descriptions because the practitioner can easily observe the necessary details in the photographs. In addition, because there are a few repeated forms, under each of those photographs will appear numbers in parenthesis which indicate the number where the original description may be found.

For the purposes of indicating the direction of movement, Chinese martial books use a compass system. The original direction which a person faces is immediately and *permanently* designated N or North for the duration of the sequence. It does not matter which actual geographic direction the individual faces, the front will always be N. From this designation, the right side becomes E or East, the left side W or West, and back side S or South.

Finally, as a last reminder, the breathing during the sequence must be smooth and fluid. Never hold the breath. Every inhalation and exhalation should last the length of the form for which it was indicated.

Yang's Barehand Tai Chi Sequence (Appendix A)

1. Beginning (T'ai-Chi Shih)

Figure 53: (N) Feet are slightly spread beyond shoulder width. Hands are at the waist, palms down. Wrists must be loose. Breathe in and out.

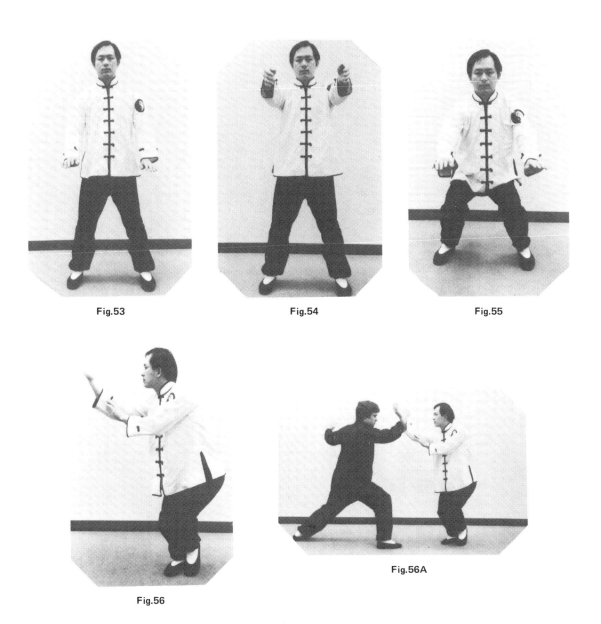

Fig.53

Fig.54

Fig.55

Fig.56

Fig.56A

Figure 54: (N) Move the wrists so the palms face each other. Lift the arms up to shoulder height. Do not raise or make the shoulders tight. Breathe in.

Figure 55: (N) Point the palms down. Move down slowly into Ma Bu. Lower the arms to knee level. Breathe out.

2. Grasp the Sparrow's Tail: Right (Yu Lan Ch'iao Wei)

Figure 56: (E) Raise the right arm, palm facing in. Bring the left leg to the right leg: left leg is on its toes. The body turns 90 degrees clockwise. Inhale. The form name describes a person gently holding a sparrow while stroking its tail.

Figure 56A: As the opponent punches, the punch is made to slide up and away.

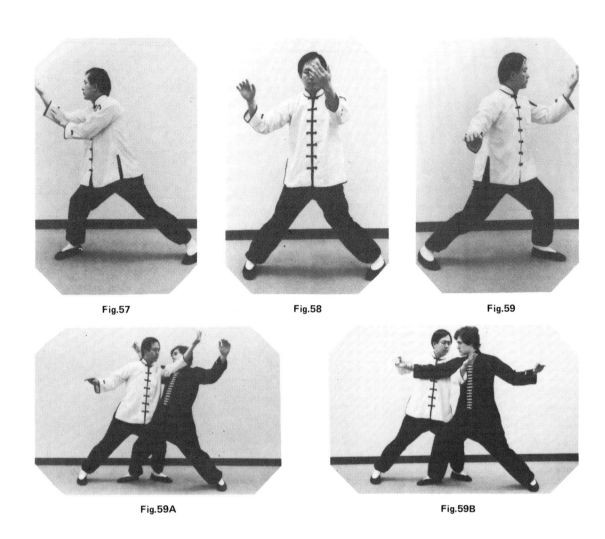

Fig.57   Fig.58   Fig.59

Fig.59A   Fig.59B

3. Grasp the Sparrow's Tail: Left (Tso Lan Ch'iao Wei)

Figure 57: (E) Transition form. Step back with your left leg. Begin to breathe out.

Figure 58: (N) Transition form. Turn on the heels into Ma Bu. Turn your left palm in, brushing by the face. Your right palm turns down. Continue to breathe out.

Figure 59: (W) Turn on the heels to W into Deng San Bu. Swing your left arm to the front and the right hand to the side, with the palms pointed down. Complete exhalation.

Figure 59A: If after blocking in 56A, the opponent withdraws his attacking arm, then the defender will step in and strike the chest.

Figure 59B: Another option after 56A: The defender grabs the punching arm, steps in, and attacks the chest muscle via a strike under the opponent's arm. In 59A and 59B, the left leg locks in back of the opponent. Even though the block and attack forms are on opposite sides in the sequence, the basic formula is still the same. Defense and attack forms, in this case, are opposite each other only to enhance the general beauty of the sequence. Only some techniques in the sequence are like this. In addition, this is a "sealing the breath" strike.

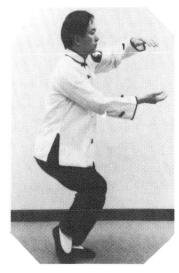

Fig.60

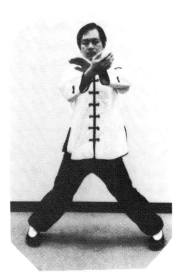

Fig.60A

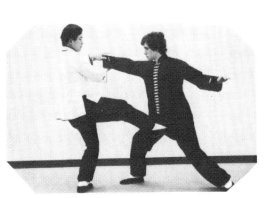

Fig.60B

Fig.61

4. Ward-Off (P'eng)

Figure 60: (W) Bring the right toe up. Swing the right hand to the front of the body, turn the palm up. The left palm turns down. Breathe in.

Figure 60A: As the attacker punches, the defender turns his body and slides the punch away.

Figure 60B: After blocking, the defender may kick the groin. This is not shown in the sequence; instead, this is a hidden technique.

Figure 61: (N) Transition form. Step back with the right leg. Turn on the heels to N while shifting into Ma Bu and crossing the hands in front of the body. Begin to breathe out.

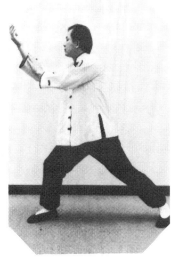

Fig.62

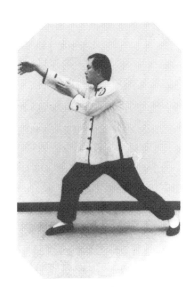

Fig.62A

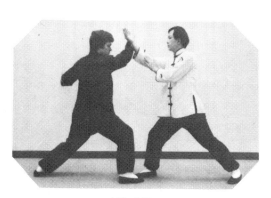

Fig.62B

Fig.63

Figure 62: (E) Turn on the heels into Deng San Bu while swinging the right arm, palms in to the front of the body. Finish exhaling.

Figure 62A: After blocking in 60A, the defender steps in and attacks the chest muscle. This is a sealing the breath technique.

Figure 62B: This form is also used as a block for the next technique.

5. Roll back (Lu)

Figure 63: (E) Extend the right arm while turning the fingers forward. Begin to inhale.

Figure 64: (E) Sit back into Ssu Lieu Bu. Move the right arm down. Left hand is at the waist. Complete inhalation.

Figure 64A: After blocking in 62A, the defender draws the opponent's hand down.

Figure 65: (E) Turn the hips slightly back. Make a gentle clockwise circle to the back of the body with your left hand. This movement does not have a practical application; instead, it is the signature of Yang's style of Tai Chi Chuan. Exhale.

6. Press (Ghi)

Figure 66: (E) Bring the left hand to the inner wrist of the right hand. Shift into Deng San Bu and extend both hands forward while still touching. Inhale when the left hand comes to the right hand. Exhale as the arms are extended.

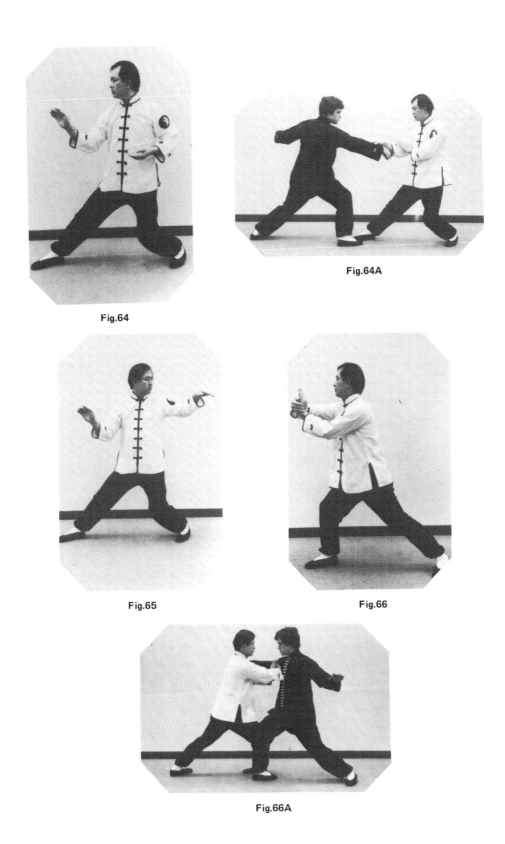

Fig.64

Fig.64A

Fig.65

Fig.66

Fig.66A

Figure 66A: After drawing in the opponent's arm, the defender strikes forward with the back of the right wrist.

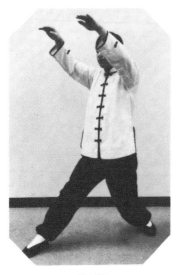

Fig.67

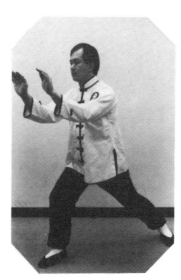

Fig.67A

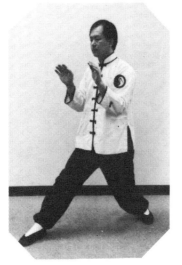

Fig.68

Fig.69

7. Push (An)

Figure 67: (E) Slide the left hand over the right hand. Open the arms so the palms face out. Sit back in Ssu Lieu Bu while raising the arms back in a circular motion. Start to breathe in.

Figure 67A: (E) As the opponent double punches, the defender slides the attacker's power up.

Figure 68: (E) Lower the arms to the chest in a circular motion. Complete inhalation.

Figure 69: (E) Shift to Deng San Bu and push the hands forward. Breathe out.

Figure 69A: Once the attacker's power is dissolved, then the defender strikes with the palms.

8. Single Whip (Tan Pien)

Figure 70: (N) Keep the arms locked in the same position and turn to N on the heels so the stance is Ma Bu. Arms swing with the body. Begin to inhale.

Figure 70A: The defender slides a punch away.

Figure 71: (W) Turn on the heels into Deng San Bu and lower the left arm, palm up. Complete inhalation.

Figure 72: (N) Bring the left leg, on its toes, to the right leg. Swing the right arm back. All the fingertips of the right hand are touching and pointing down. Exhale.

Figure 72A: The defender slides an opponent's punch away. Fingertips touch so the attacker's hand is hooked. This form is also used to block and slide away an opponent's long weapon, such as a rod.

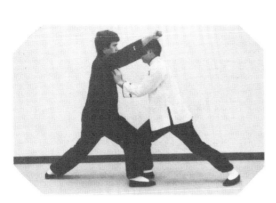

Fig.69A

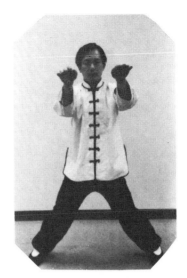

Fig.70

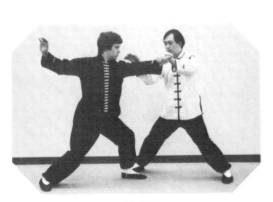

Fig.70A

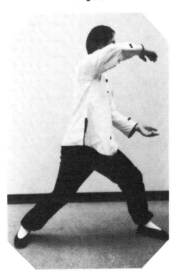

Fig.71

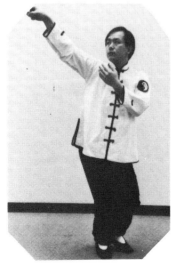

Fig.72

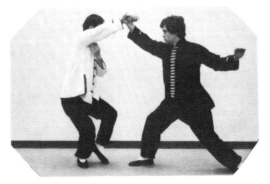

Fig.72A

45

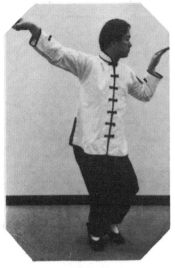

Fig.73

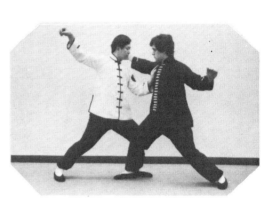

Fig.73A

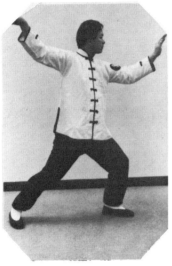

Fig.74

Fig.74A

Figure 73: (W) Turn the body to face W. At the same time move the left hand across the body, palm pointed in. Next, turn the palm out. Inhale.

Figure 73A: After blocking, the left hand circles the punching arm and pushes it to the side.

Figure 74: (W) Step the left leg forward so the stance is Deng San Bu, and push the left hand forward. Exhale.

Figure 74A: The defender strikes the opponent's chest.

9. Lift Hands and Lean Forward (T'i Shou Shang Shih)

Figure 75: (N) Bring the right leg up to the left. Drop the hands down and bring them up to the chest. Inhale.

Figure 76: (N) Lift the right knee up with the arms. Place the right leg down on its heel. At the same time, extend the right hand forward, fingers pointing to the front. Exhale.

Figure 76A: As the opponent punches, the defender slides the attack up, then kicks the knee.

10. The Crane Spreads Its Wings (Pai Hao Liang Ch'ih)

Figure 77: (W) Set the right foot down. Turn the body to W and into Ma Bu; simultaneously, swing the right arm down and up, making it cross the left hand which has remained stationary. Both feet are parallel.

Figure 78: (W) Spread the arms, right arm higher than the left, while bringing the left leg to the right leg; the left leg has its toes slightly off the floor. As the arms are spread, lean slightly to the right side while pointing the right foot out 45 degrees. Lift the left leg and set it down on its toes. Exhale. The arms are the wings being spread open.

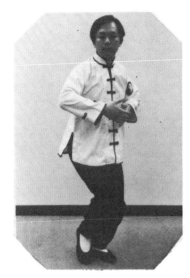

Fig.75

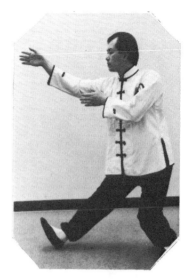

Fig.76

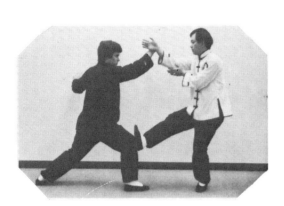

Fig.76A

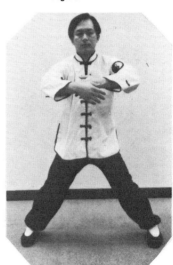

Fig.77

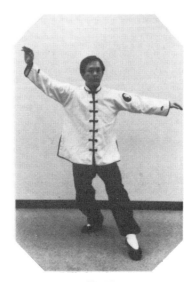

Fig.78

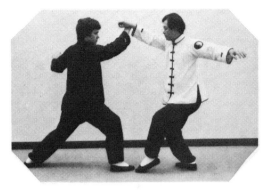

Fig.78A

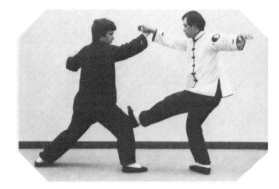

Fig.78B

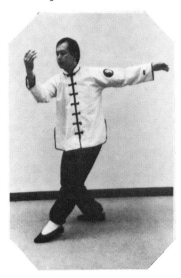

Fig.79

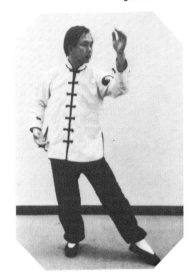

Fig.80

Figure 78A: As the attacker punches, the defender's right hand slides the fist away.

Figure 78B: The next move may be to kick the attacker's leg. This technique or application is not shown or performed in the sequence.

11. Brush Knee and Step Forward: Left (Tso Lou Hsi Yao Pu)

Figure 79: (W) Swing the right arm across the body and then down to the waist. Inhale.

Figure 80: (W) Swing the left arm across the body. Exhale.

Figure 80A: The Defender blocks the attacker's punch.

Figure 80B: The defender may kick the opponent's knee after blocking.

Figure 81: (W) As the left hand reaches the center of the body, raise the left knee, swing the left arm past it, and raise the right arm back and up. Complete exhalation.

Figure 81A: As the attacker kicks, the defender slides the leg away while also hooking it.

Figure 82: (W) Step down with the left leg into Deng San Bu. Inhale. Push forward with the right palm. Exhale.

Figure 82A: After blocking the kick, the defender moves in to strike.

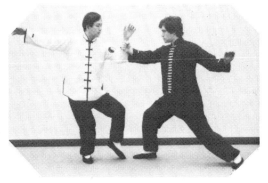

Fig.80A

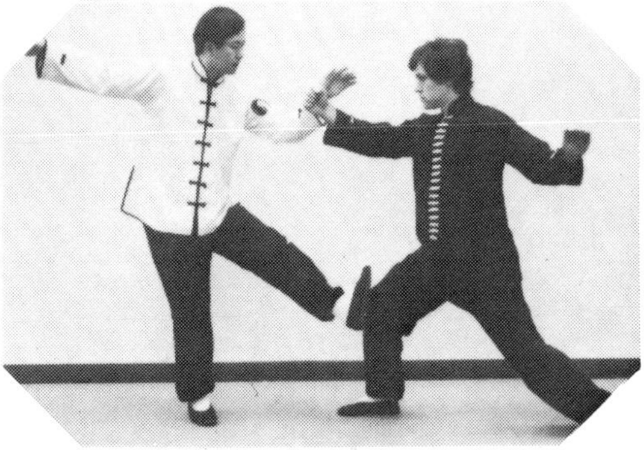

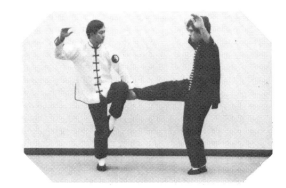

Fig.80B

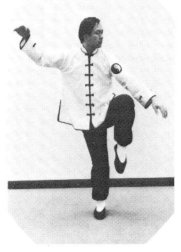

Fig.81

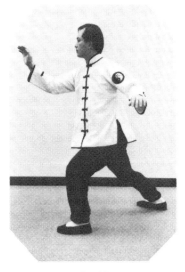

Fig.81A

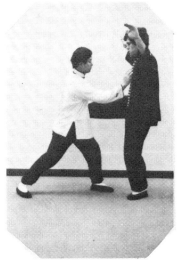

Fig.82

Fig.82A

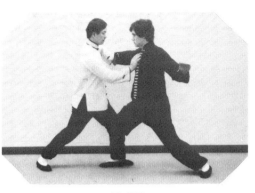

Fig.82B

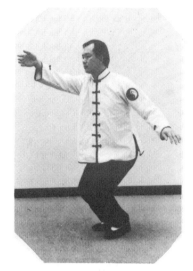

Fig.83

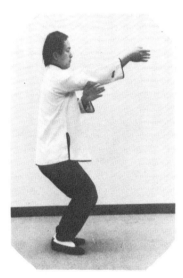

Fig.84

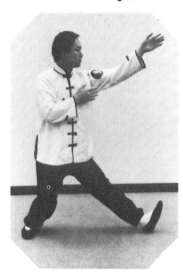

Fig.85

Figure 82B: If the attacker blocked as in 80A, then the defender moves in to hit the chest.

12. Play the Guitar (Shou Hui P'i P'a)

Figure 83: (W) Bring the right leg up with the knee lifted. Turn the right palm to the side. Step down with the right leg. Inhale.

Figure 84: (W) Put the back of the left hand on the outside portion of the right arm and lift the left knee. Begin to exhale.

Figure 85: (W) Slide the left hand forward along the right arm. Put the left leg down on its heel. Extend the left hand, palm to the side and fingers pointing forward. Exhale. The left hand holds the guitar, while the right plays it. Complete exhalation.

Figure 85A: The defender blocks a punch, then kicks the knee of the opponent.

13. Brush Knee and Step Forward: Left (Tso Lou Hsi Yao Pu)

Figures 86 (W), 87 (W), 88(W). Repeat No. 11.

14. Brush Knee and Step Forward: Right (Yu Lou Hsi Yao Pu)

Figure 89: (W) Make a counterclockwise circle with the left arm. Turn the left foot so the stance is Dsao Pan. The right foot is on its toe. Inhale.

Figure 89A: The defender blocks the punch and turns his body.

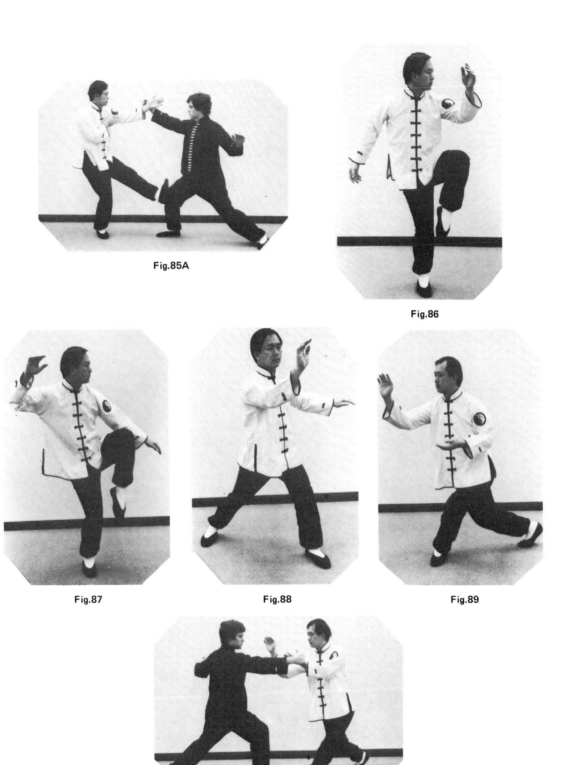

Fig.85A

Fig.86

Fig.87

Fig.88

Fig.89

Fig.89A

51

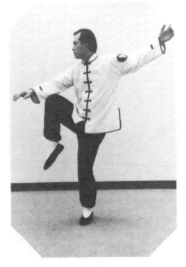

Fig.90

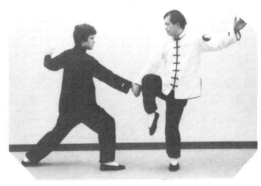

Fig.90A

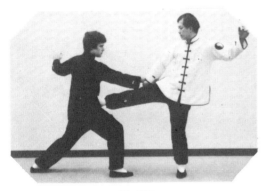

Fig.90B

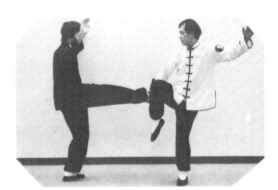

Fig.90C

Figure 90: (W) Raise the right knee while swinging the right hand in front of it. The arm swings back and up. Exhale.

Figure 90A: The defender swings the blocked arm down; or the defender can block a low punch.

Figure 90B: After blocking the arm, the defender can kick. This application is not performed in the sequence.

Figure 90C: The left hand of the defender may also block a kick.

Figure 91: (W) Step down with the right leg. Inhale. Push forward with the left palm. Exhale.

Figure 91A: After blocking the kick in 90C, the defender strikes in.

Figure 91B: If a punch is blocked by the defender, then he pushes the arm away and attacks the opponent's back.

15. Brush Knee and Step Forward: Left (Tso Lou Hsi Yao Pu)

Figure 92: (W) Make a clockwise circle with the hand and shift into Dsao Pan Bu. Inhale.

Figures 93: (W), 94 (W). Repeat No. 11.

16. Play the Guitar (Shou Hui P'i P'a)

Figures 95 (W), 96 (W), 97 (W). Repeat No. 12.

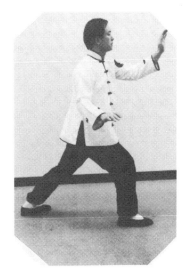

Fig.91

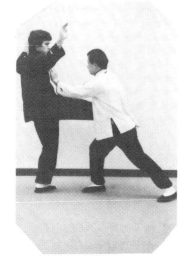

Fig.91A

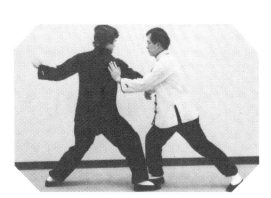

Fig.91B

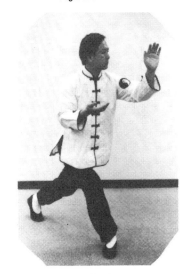

Fig.92

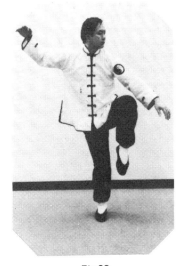

Fig.93

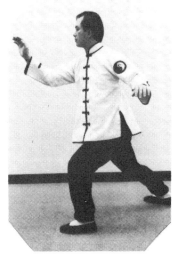

Fig.94

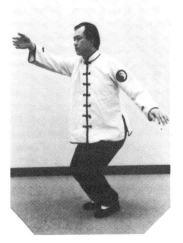

Fig.95

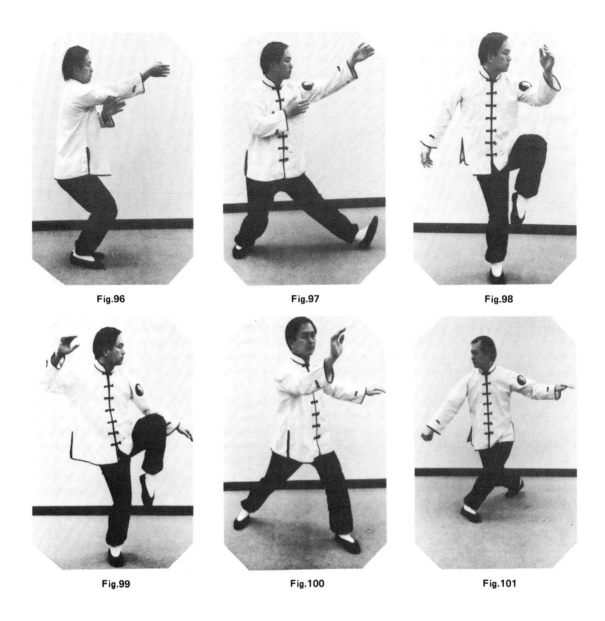

Fig.96	Fig.97	Fig.98
Fig.99	Fig.100	Fig.101

17. Brush Knee and Step Forward: Left (Tso Lou Hsi Yao Pu)
Figures 98 (W), 99 (W), 100 (W). Repeat No. 11.

18. Twist Body and Circle Fist (Pieh Shen Ch'ui)
Figure 101: (W) Shift the stance to Dsao Pan Bu while the right arm, in a fist, makes a big semi-circle from the front of the chest down to the thighs. Start to inhale.

19. Step Forward, Deflect Downward, Parry and Punch (Chin Pu Pan Lan Ch'ui)
Figure 102: (W) Step forward with the right leg into Dsao Pan Bu while circling the right arm up and then to the waist. The left arm swings across the body. Complete inhalation.

Figure 102A: As the opponent punches, the defender deflects the punch. This form may also be used as an upward strike with the form in 101 as the block.

Figure 102B: After 102A, the opponent's arm is controlled by the defender's left hand and deflected down.

Figure 103: (W) Step forward with the left leg into Deng San Bu and punch. Exhale.

Figure 103A: The opponent's arm is pushed to the side while he steps in to attack.

20. Seal Tightly (Ju Feng Ssu Pi)
Figure 104: (W) Put the left palm under the elbow. Start to breathe in.

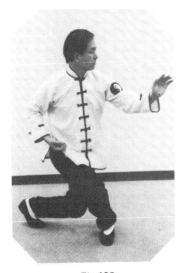

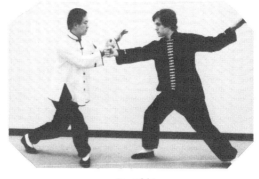

Fig.102A

Fig.102

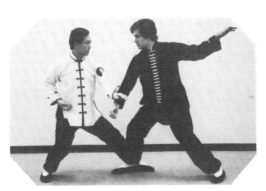

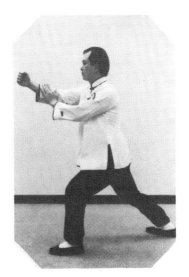

Fig.102B

Fig.103

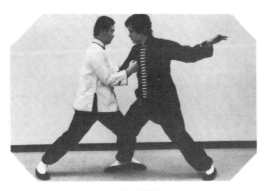

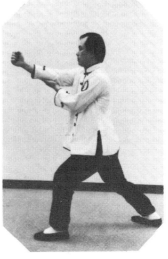

Fig.103A

Fig.104

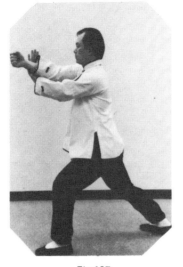

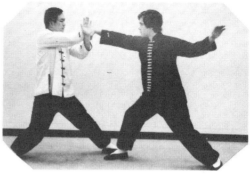

Fig.105A

Fig.105

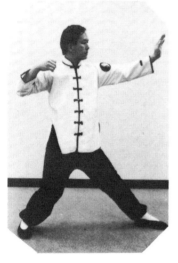

Fig.106

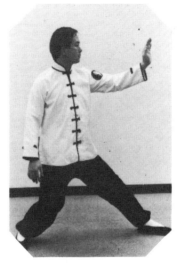

Fig.107

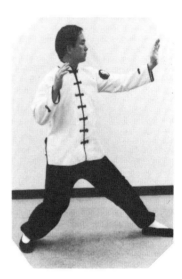

Fig.108

Figure 105: (W) Twist the palm so the back of the left hand is touching the outside portion of the right arm. Slide the left hand forward. Continue to inhale.

Figure 105A: An opponent grabs the defender's right wrist. The defender slides the hand forward to release himself.

Figure 106: (W) Withdraw the right arm to the rear while sitting back in Ssu Lieu Bu. Complete inhalation.

Figure 107: (W) Drop the right arm down. Exhale.

Figure 108: (W) Raise the right arm up so it is behind the ear. Inhale.

Figure 109: (W) Shift the stance to Deng San Bu and push the right palm forward. Exhale.

Figure 109A: After releasing his arm, the defender strikes forward.

21. Embrace the Tiger and Return to the Mountain (Pao Hu Guei Shan)

Figure 110: (N) Cross the hands and turn the body N. Lean to the right side. Inhale.

Figure 110A: The Defender deflects the opponent's punch up.

Figure 111: (N) Squat down into Fu Hu Bu while circling both arms out, down, and in. Weight is on the right leg. Begin to exhale.

Figure 111A: After blocking, the defender moves in to attack the groin. Continue exhaling.

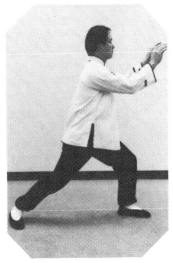

Fig.109

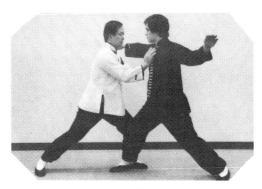

Fig.109A

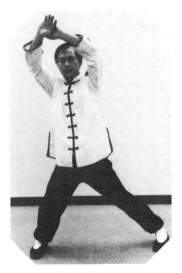

Fig.110

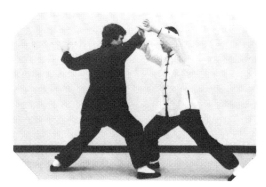

Fig.110A

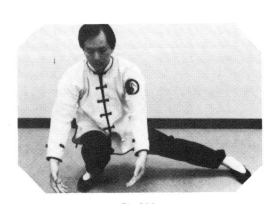

Fig.111

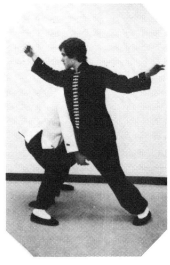

Fig.111A

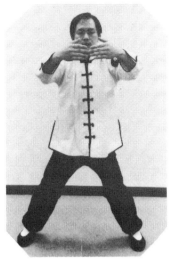

Fig.112

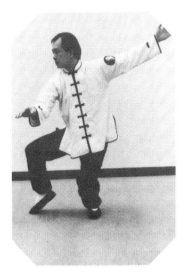

Fig.113

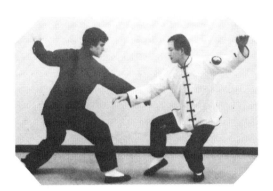

Fig.113A

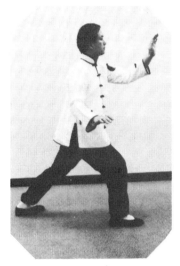

Fig.114

22. Close Tai Chi (Ho T'ai-Chi)

Figure 112: (N) Shift the weight to the left leg, raise the right knee, and step the right leg down in Ma Bu. Arms are in a circle. Complete exhaling.

23. Ward-Off, Rollback, Press, and Push (P'eng Lu Ghi An)

Figure 113: (E) Raise the right leg on its toe. Swing the right arm down; the left arm comes up. Inhale.

Figure 113A: The defender blocks a punch.

Figure 114: (E) Shift into Deng San Bu, right leg forward, and push the left hand forward. Exhale.

Figure 114A: After blocking and sliding the punch away, the defender strikes the opponent's back.

Figure 115: (N) Keep the arms in the same position and turn 180 degrees on the heels. Start to inhale.

Figures 116 (W), 117 (N), 118 (E), 119 (E), 120 (E), 121 (E), 122 (E), 123 (E), 124 (E), 125 (E). Repeat Nos. 4, 5, 6, and 7.

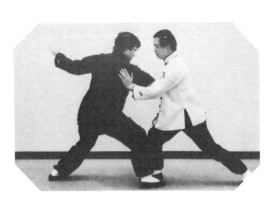

Fig.114A

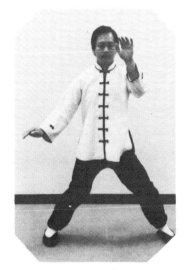

Fig.115

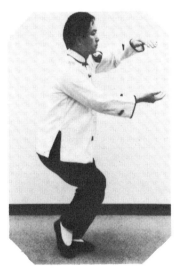

Fig.116

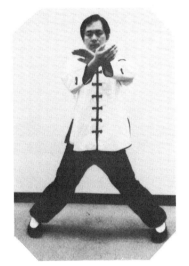

Fig.117

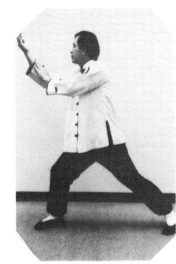

Fig.118

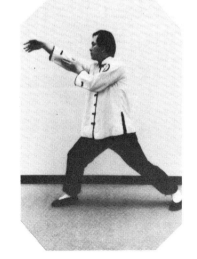

Fig.119

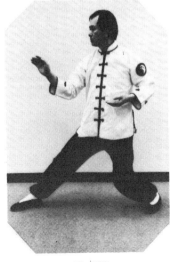

Fig.120

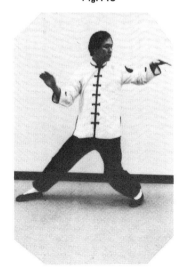

Fig.121

59

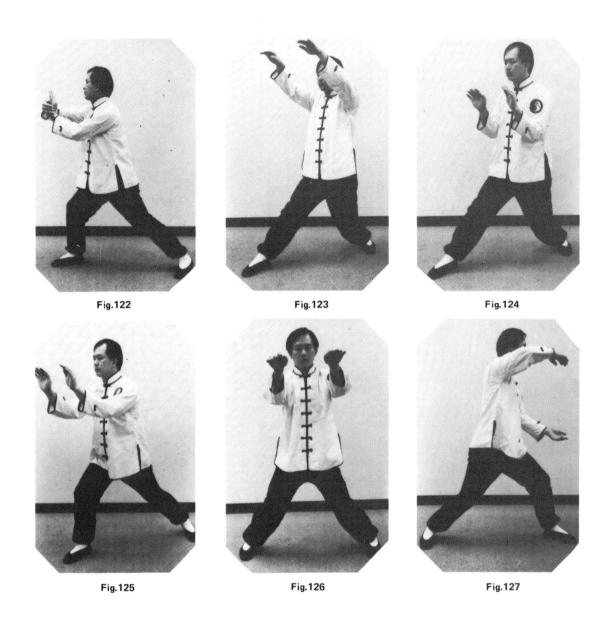

Fig.122   Fig.123   Fig.124

Fig.125   Fig.126   Fig.127

24. Single Whip (Tan Pien)

Figures 126 (N), 127 (W), 128 (N), 129 (W), 130 (W). Repeat No. 8.

25. Punch Under the Elbow (Chou Ti K'an Ch'ui)

Figure 131: (W) Bring the right foot, on its toes, up to the left leg while moving the right hand over the head. Begin to breathe in.

Figure 132: (N) Step to N with the right leg. Complete inhalation.

Figure 133: (W) Turn the body W, raise the left leg, and move the right arm down and in front of the body. The left hand then moves up on the inside of the right arm. Begin to breathe out.

Figure 133A: The defender blocks a punch from the inside position.

Figures 134: (W) Set the left foot down on the heel while bringing the left elbow up above the right fist. Complete exhalation.

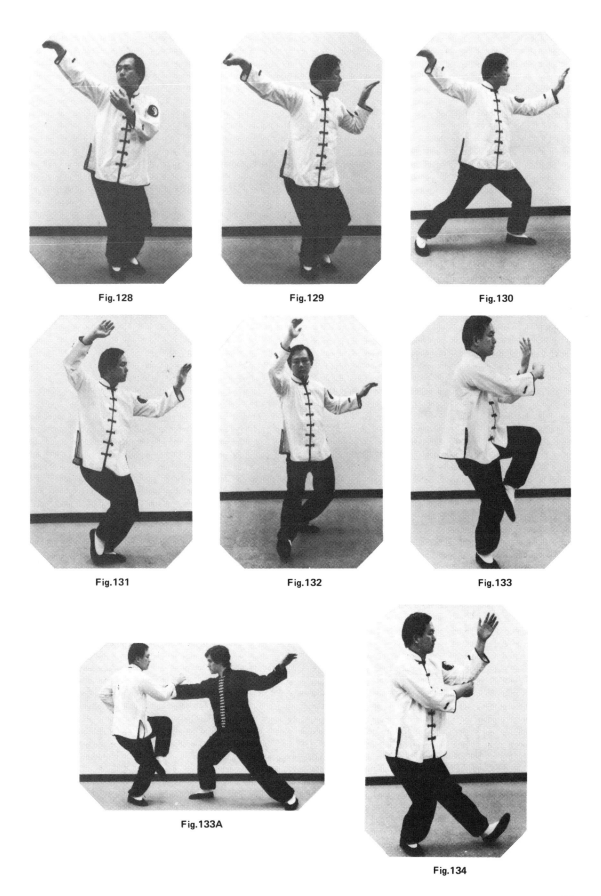

Fig.128

Fig.129

Fig.130

Fig.131

Fig.132

Fig.133

Fig.133A

Fig.134

61

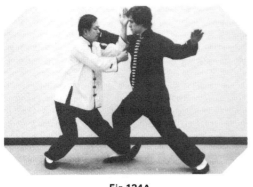

Fig.134A

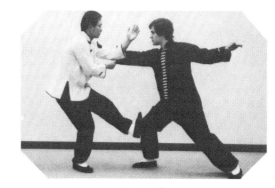

Fig.134B

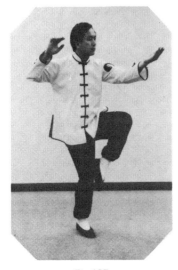

Fig.135

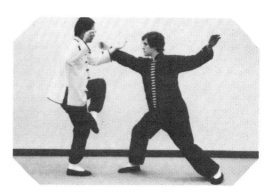

Fig.135A

Figure 134A: The defender attacks with the left hand while locking the opponent's right leg.

Figure 134B: The defender may also kick the attacker's knee.

26. Step Back and Repulse Monkey: Left (Tso Tao Nien Hou)

Figure 135: (W) Raise the left knee. Make a counterclockwise circle with the left hand so the palm ends facing up. Swing the right hand down, back, and up so the palm faces forward. Begin inhalation.

Figure 135A: As the opponent punches, the defender blocks to the side.

Figure 135B: The defender may then kick the attacker. Not shown in sequence.

Figure 136: (W) Turn on your right heel slightly and extend the left leg back. Attempt to make your leg horizontal to ground. Exhale.

Figure 137: (W) Step down with the left leg and complete exhalation. Shift into Ssu Lieu Bu while pushing forward with the right palm, withdrawing the left palm to the waist.

Figure 137A: After blocking, the chest is attacked.

27. Step Back and Repulse Monkey: Right (Yu Tao Nien Hou)

Figure 138: (W) Lift the right knee up. Make a clockwise circle with the right hand, palm up. Swing the left hand down, back, and up so the palm faces front. Begin inhalation.

Figure 138A: The defender blocks the punch from the outside.

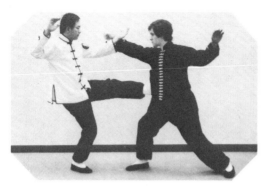

Fig.135B

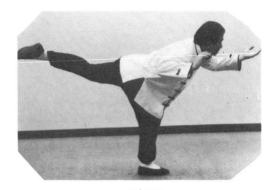

Fig.136

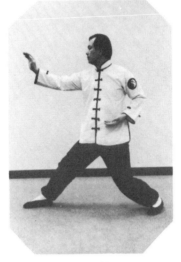

Fig.137

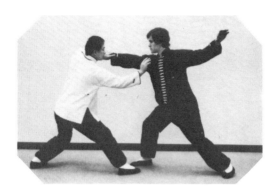

Fig.137A

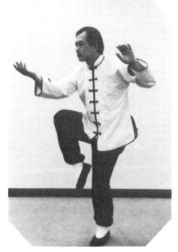

Fig.138

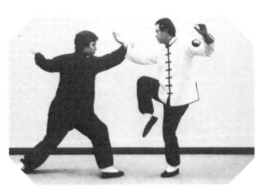

Fig138A

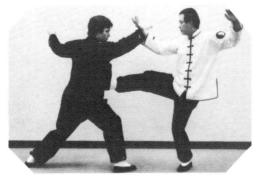

Fig.138B

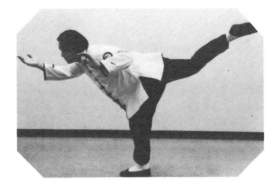

Fig.139

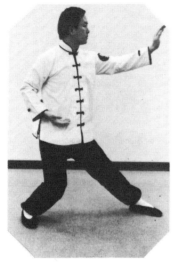

Fig.140

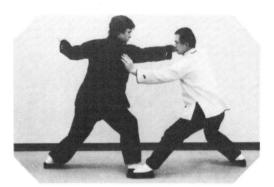

Fig.140B

Figure 138B: Next, the defender may kick. Not shown in sequence.

Figure 139: (W) Turn slightly on the left heel and extend the right leg back. Begin exhalation.

Figure 140: (W) Step down with the right leg and complete exhalation. Shift into Ssu Lieu Bu while pushing the left palm forward and retreating the right palm to the waist.

Figure 140A: The defender strikes the opponent's back.

28. Step Back and Repulse Monkey: Left (Tso Tao Nien Hou)

Figures 141 (W), 142 (W), 143 (W). Repeat No. 26.

29. Diagonal Flying (Hsieh Fei Shih)

Figure 144: (S) Move the left hand up and the right hand down. Same as 60. Inhale.

Figure 144A: The defender blocks the punch to the side.

Figure 145: (N) Turn 180 degrees clockwise on the left heel. Step the right leg down into Deng San Bu while sliding the right hand, palm up, to the front of the face. The left hand moves down to the side. Exhale.

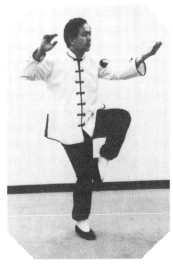

Fig.141

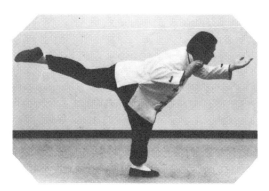

Fig.142

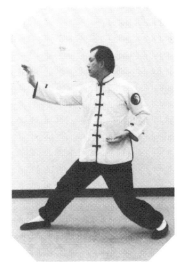

Fig.143

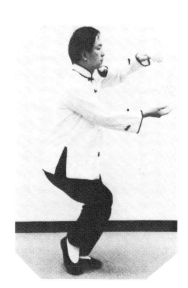

Fig.144

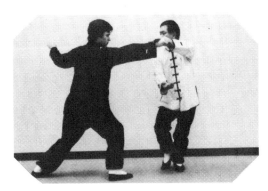

Fig.144A

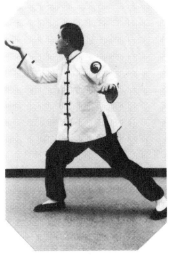

Fig.145

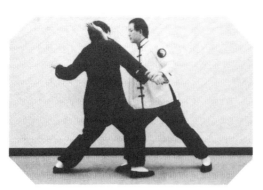

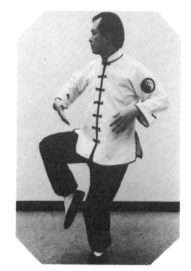

Fig.145A

Fig.146

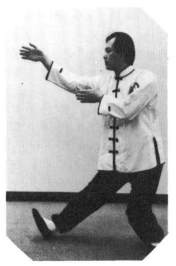

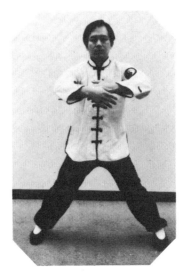

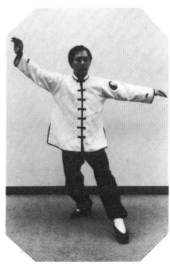

Fig.147

Fig.148

Fig.149

Figure 145A: After blocking, the defender attacks the side of the neck with the forearm.

30. Lift the Hands and Lean Forward (T'i Shou Shang Shih)

Figure 146: (N) Slide the right knee up and the arms in. Inhale.

Figure 147: (W) Repeat No. 9.

31. The Crane Spreads Its Wings (Pai Hao Liang Ch'ih)

Figures 148 (W), 149 (W). Repeat No. 10.

32. Brush Knee and Step Forward: Left (Tso Lou Hsi Yao Pu)

Figures 150 (W), 151 (W), 152 (W), 153 (W). Repeat No. 11.

33. Pick Up the Needle from the Sea Bottom (Hai Ti Lao Chen)

Figure 154: (W) Withdraw the left leg in on its toes while bringing the right hand back, palm facing in, and pushing out the left palm. Inhale.

Figure 154A: As the opponent strikes, the defender slides the punch up with both arms. The left hand may attack the elbow.

Figure 155: (W) Scoop down, the right hand "picking" an object from the floor. Exhale.

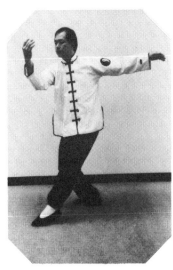

Fig.150

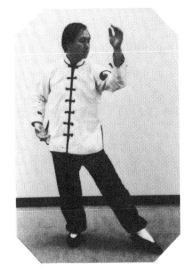

Fig.151

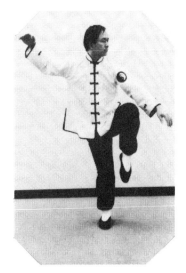

Fig.152

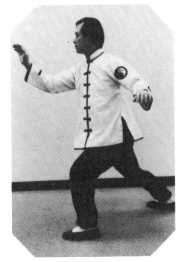

Fig.153

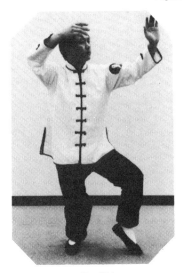

Fig.154

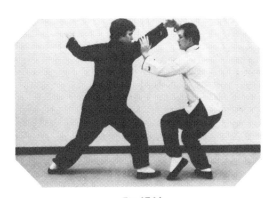

Fig.154A

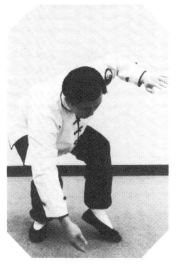

Fig.155

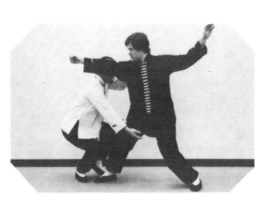

Fig.155A

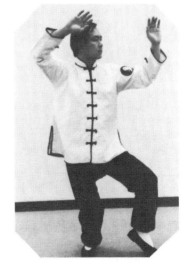

Fig.156

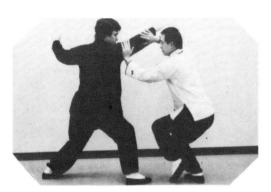

Fig.156A

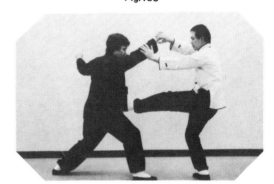

Fig.156B

Figure 155A: After blocking, the defender stoops low to attack the groin. In China, the head was considered to be the heaven and the groin area the sea. Picking a needle from the sea thus implies a groin attack.

34. Fan Back (Shan T'ung Pei)

Figure 156: (W) Stand up into the position of 154 but with the right palm facing out. Inhale.

Figure 156A: The defender slides the punch away.

Figure 156B: The defender then may kick. Not shown in this sequence.

Figure 157: (W) Shift the stance into Deng San Bu while moving both arms forward. Exhale.

Figure 157A: After blocking, the defender pushes forward to knock his opponent off balance.

35. Turn, Twist Body, and Circle Fist (Chuan Shen Pieh Shen Ch'ui)

Figure 158: (N) Turn N into Ma Bu and circumscribe a large counterclockwise circle in front of the body with the left hand. Inhale.

Figure 159: (E) As the left hand circle nears completion, circumscribe a large clockwise circle with the right arm, in a fist, to the side of the body. Head looks E. Complete inhalation.

36. Step Forward, Deflect Downward, Parry and Punch (Chin Pu, Pan, Lan, Ch'ui)

Figure 160: (E) Turn your body in Dsao Pan Bu while withdrawing the right hand to your waist, swinging the left hand across the body. Refer to 102A for application. Start exhalation.

Figure 161: (E) Step forward with the left leg into Deng San Bu and punch with the right fist. Complete exhalation. Refer to 103A for application.

37. Step Forward, Ward-Off, Rollback, Press and Push (Shang Pu P'eng Lu Ghi An)

Figure 162: (W) Turn the legs so the stance is Dsao Pan Bu while lowering your right hand, palm up, into the Ward-Off position of 60. Inhale.

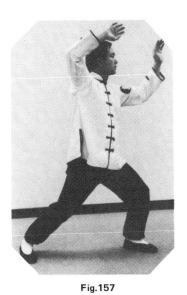

Fig.157

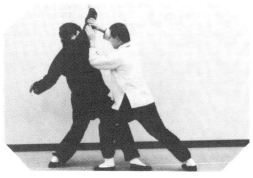

Fig.157A

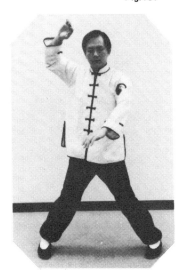

Fig.158

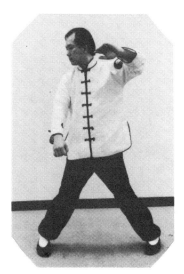

Fig.159

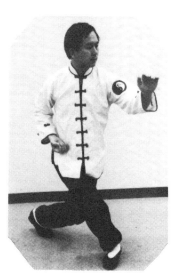

Fig.160

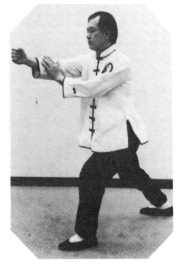

Fig.161

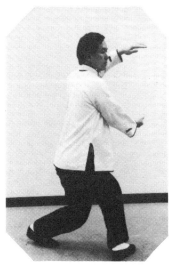

Fig.162

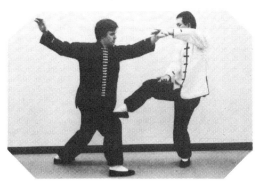

Fig.162A

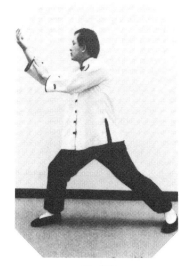

Fig.163

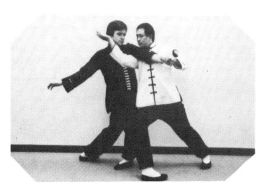

Fig.163A

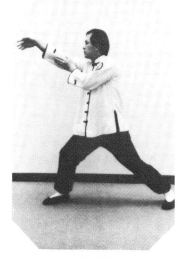

Fig.164

Figure 162A: After blocking, the martial artist may kick the opponent's groin.

Figure 163: (W) Step forward with the right leg into Deng San Bu and swing the right arm up. Exhale.

Figure 163A: After blocking, the defender steps in to strike the chest with his arm. The opponent's elbow must be flat and stiff. This form can also be used as a block.

Figures 164 (E), 165 (E), 166 (E), 167 (E), 168 (E), 169 (E) 170 (N). Repeat Nos. 4, 5, 6, and 7.

38. Single Whip (Tan Pien)

Figures 171 (W), 172 (W), 173 (W), 174 (W), 175 (W). Repeat No. 8.

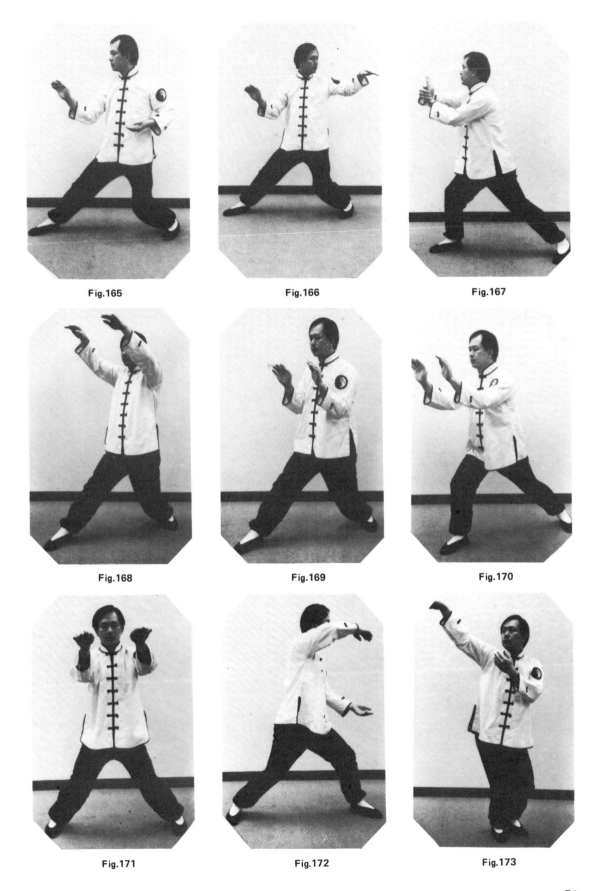

Fig.165　　　　　　　　Fig.166　　　　　　　　Fig.167

Fig.168　　　　　　　　Fig.169　　　　　　　　Fig.170

Fig.171　　　　　　　　Fig.172　　　　　　　　Fig.173

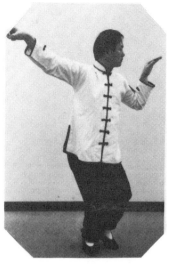

Fig. 174

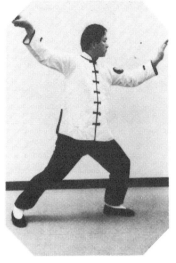

Fig. 175

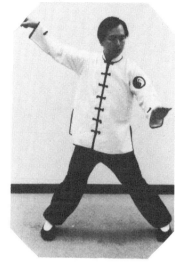

Fig. 176

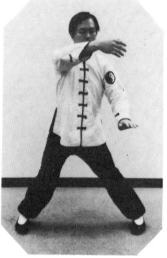

Fig. 177

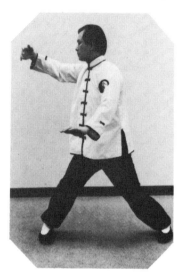

Fig. 178

39. Wave Hand in the Clouds: Right (Yu Yun Shou)

Figure 176: (N) Turn N into Ma Bu while dropping the left hand down. Start inhalation.

Figure 177: (N) Swing the right arm, palm facing your body, down and up so it passes directly in front of the left hand. Move the right arm up until shoulder height and above the left hand. Complete inhalation.

Figure 178: (N) Turn the upper body to the right side while keeping the arms locked. The arms will turn with the body. Exhale.

Figure 178A: As an opponent punches, the defender guides the attacking power to the side.

40. Wave Hands in the Clouds: Left (Tso Yun Shou)

Figure 179: (N) Bring the left leg to the right leg. Turn the right palm to the ground while moving the right arm straight down; at same time, turn the left palm in while moving the left arm straight up. Inhale.

Figure 179A: The defender hooks his opponent's arm in order to pull.

Figure 180: (E) Turn the upper body to the left side. Exhale.

41. Wave Hands in the Clouds: Right (Yu Yun Shou)

Figure 181: (N) Turn the left palm to the ground while moving the left arm down; at the same time, turn the right palm in while moving the right arm up. Step to the side with the right leg. Inhale.

Figure 182: (N) Turn the upper body into Ma Bu facing N. Start exhalation.

Figure 183: (E) Turn the upper body to right. Complete exhalation.

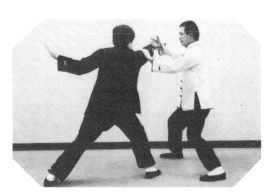

Fig.178A

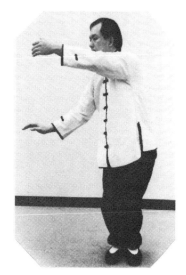

Fig.179

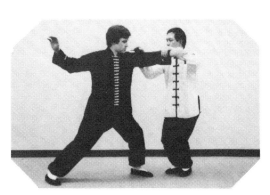

Fig.179A

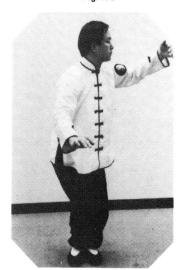

Fig.180

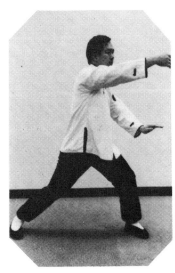

Fig.181

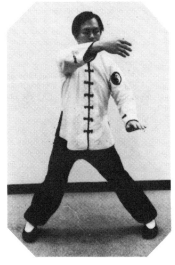

Fig.182

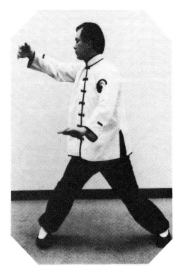

Fig.183

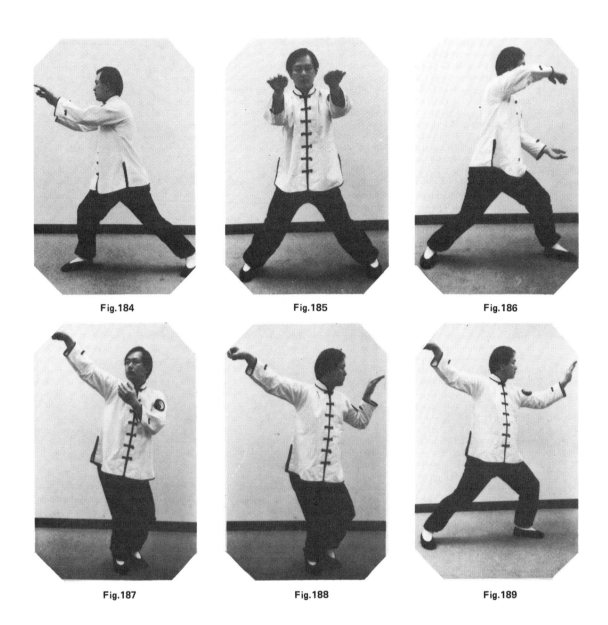

Fig.184   Fig.185   Fig.186

Fig.187   Fig.188   Fig.189

42. Single Whip (Tan Pien)

Figure 184: (N) Shift to Deng San Bu while raising both hands up. Begin to breathe in.

Figures 185 (W), 186 (N), 187 (W), 188 (W), 189 (W). Repeat No. 8.

43. Stand High to Search Out the Horse (Kao T'an Ma)

Figure 190: (W) Bring the left leg back on its toe while opening both hands and raising them up slightly. Begin to breathe in. Application is the same as 156A and B.

44. Separate Right Foot (Yu Fen Chiao)

Figure 191: (W) Pick up the left knee and then set the left foot down into Dsao Pan Bu. Breathe out. Cross your hands to the side of your body, palms face in. Inhale.

Figure 191A: As an opponent punches, the defender sweeps the punch away.

Figure 192: (W) Open up both arms, palms out, and snap kick the right leg so it touches the right palm. Exhale.

Figure 192A: After sweeping the punch away, the defender kicks.

45. Separate Left Foot (Tso Fen Chiao)

Figure 193: (W) Step the right leg down so the stance is Dsao Pan Bu and cross your arms to the side of the body, palms in. Inhale.

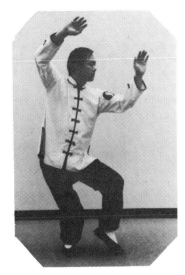

Fig.190

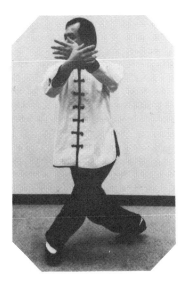

Fig.191

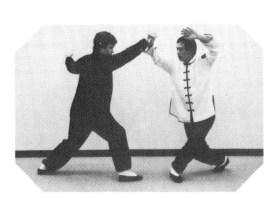

Fig.191A

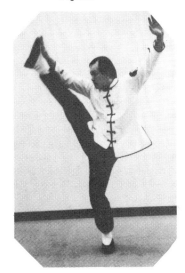

Fig.192

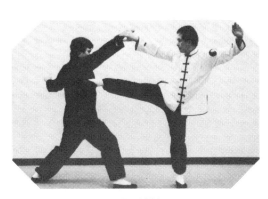

Fig.192A

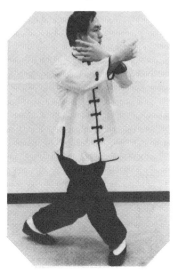

Fig.193

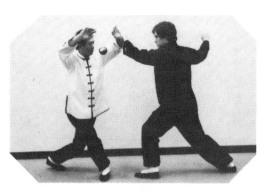

Fig.193A

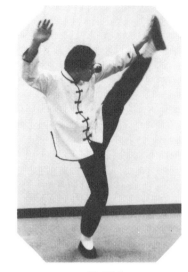

Fig.194

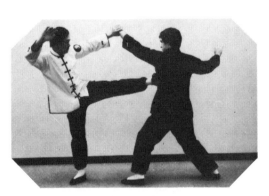

Fig.194A

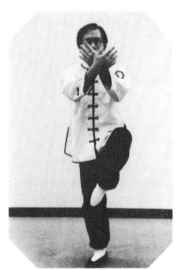

Fig.195

Figure 193A: The defender blocks the punch.

Figure 194: (W) Open both arms, palms out, and snap kick the left leg so it touches the left palm. Exhale.

46. Turn and Kick with Heel (90 degrees) (Chuan Shen Teng Chiao)

Figure 195: (S) Bring the left leg in so its knee is raised. Do not let the left leg touch the ground after the kick. Cross your hands in front of the body. Inhale.

Figure 196: (S) Spin 90 degrees counterclockwise on the right heel. Open both arms and kick with the left heel. Exhale.

Figure 196A: The defender blocks a double punch and kicks to the abdomen.

47. Brush Knee and Step Forward: Left (Tso Lou Hsi Yao Pu)

Figure 197: (S) Bring the left foot in, knee raised, and swing the right hand past the left knee while raising the right hand. Inhale.

Figure 198: (S) Repeat 82. Exhale.

48. Brush Knee and Step Forward: Right (Yu Lou Hsi Yao Pu)

Figures 199 (S), 200 (S), 201 (S). Repeat No. 14.

49. Step Forward and Strike Down with the Fist (Chin Pu Tsai Ch'ui)

Figure 202: (S) Turn the left leg so the stance is Dsao Pan Bu. Swing the left arm across the body and retreat the right hand in a fist to the waist. Inhale.

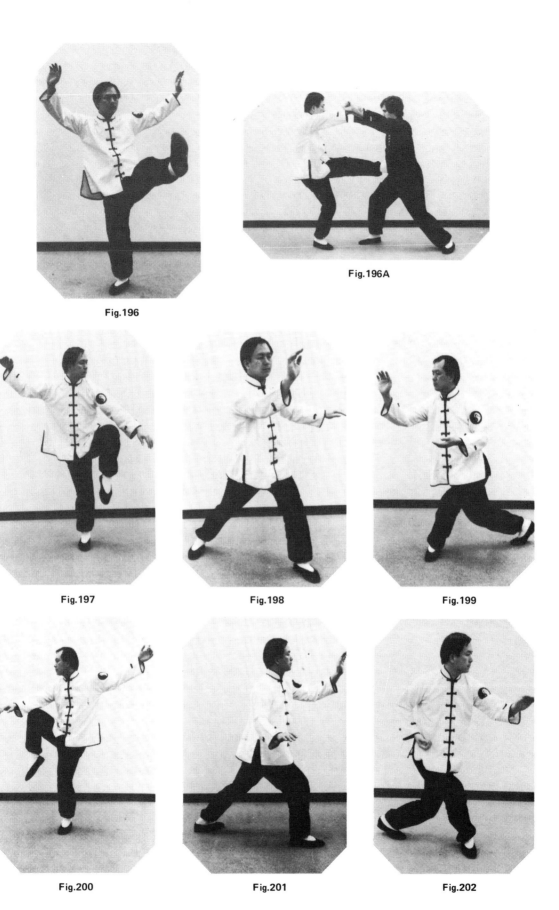

Fig.196

Fig.196A

Fig.197

Fig.198

Fig.199

Fig.200

Fig.201

Fig.202

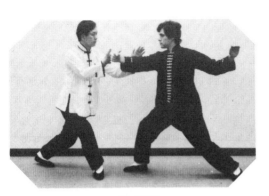

Fig.202A

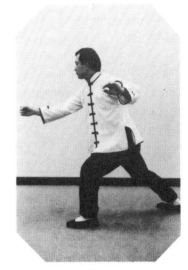

Fig.203

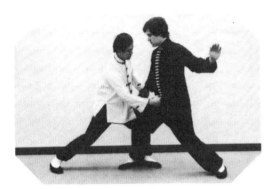

Fig.203A

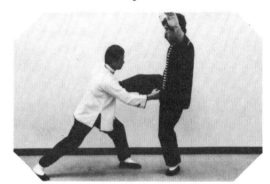

Fig.203B

Figure 202A: The defender slides the punch away.

Figure 203: (S) Step forward with the left leg while sweeping the left arm down and back across the body. Punch low so the palm of the fist is facing the side. Exhale.

Figure 203A: The defender sweeps the punching hand to the side and attacks the belly.

Figure 203B: The defender may also block a kick, then step to punch.

50. Turn and Twist the Body and Circle the Arm (Chuan Shen Pieh Shen Ch'ui)

Figure 204: (N) Turn 90 degrees clockwise into Ma Bu. Begin to inhale. The right hand circles down.

51. Step Forward, Deflect Downward, Parry and Punch (Chin Pu, Pan, Lan Ch'ui)

Figure 205: (N) Turn another 90 degrees into Dsao Pan Bu while swinging the right and left hands across the body. Complete inhalation.

Figure 206: (N) Step forward with the left leg and repeat 103. Exhale. Refer to similar forms for application.

52. Kick Right (Yu Ti Chiao)

Figure 207: (N) Turn the left leg so the stance is Dsao Pan Bu and cross your arms in front of your body. Inhale.

Figure 208: (N) Open your arms and kick with the right heel.

Figure 208A: The defender blocks high and kicks low.

53. Strike the Tiger: Right (Yu Ta Fu)

Figure 209: (N) Step down with the right leg into Deng San Bu and swing the right hand down and up. Start inhalation.

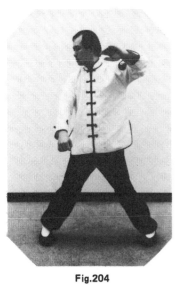
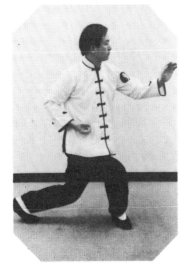
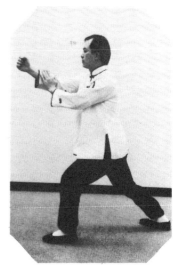

Fig.204   **Fig.205**   **Fig.206**

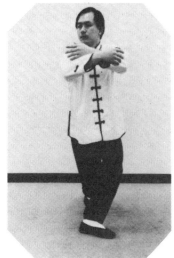
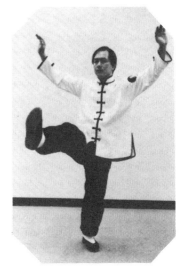

Fig.207   **Fig.208**

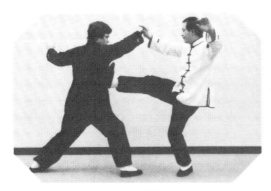
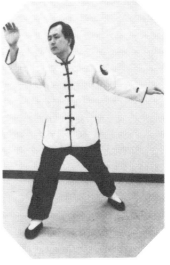

Fig.208A

Fig.209

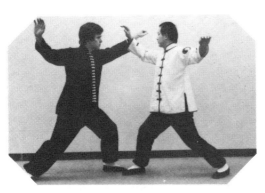

Fig.209A

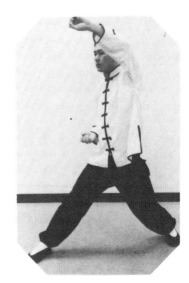

Fig.210

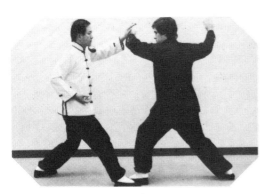

Fig.210A

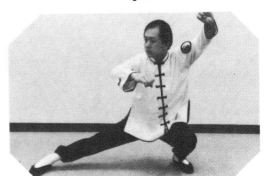

Fig.211

Figure 209A: The defender blocks the punch from the inside position.

Figure 210: (N) Slide the left hand up the right arm, then bring the right hand to the waist, and sit in Ssu Lieu Bu. The left arm remains extended. Complete inhalation.

Figure 210A: After blocking, the defender slides his left arm to the outside of the attacker's punch.

Figure 211: (W) Change the stance to Fu Hu Bu, weight on the left leg. Hook the right fist across the body. The left arm remains up. Exhale.

Figure 211A: The defender pulls on the attacker's arm and punches the opponent's side.

Figure 211B: The defender may also strike the side of the head.

54. Strike the Tiger: Left (Tso Ta Fu)

Figure 212: (W) Move the right hand under the left elbow. Slide the right arm up the left forearm. Begin to inhale.

Figure 213: (W) Bring the left fist to the waist while the right hand swings up. Complete inhalation. Shift weight to the right leg, remaining in the Fu Hu Bu posture. Hook the left fist across the body. Exhale.

Figure 213A: This is the opposite of the Strike the Tiger: Right form. The defender blocks with the left hand, the right hand slides the punch away, then pulls and strikes the opponent's side.

Figure 213B: The defender may also strike the side of the head.

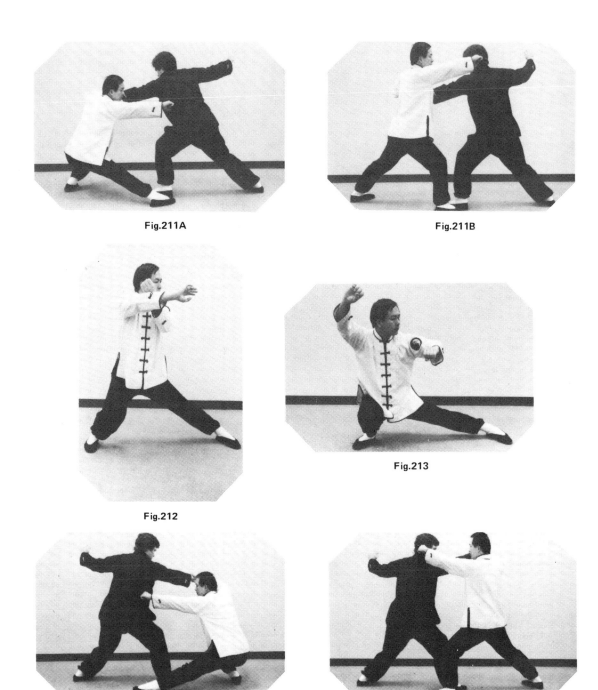

Fig.211A

Fig.211B

Fig.212

Fig.213

Fig.213A

Fig.213B

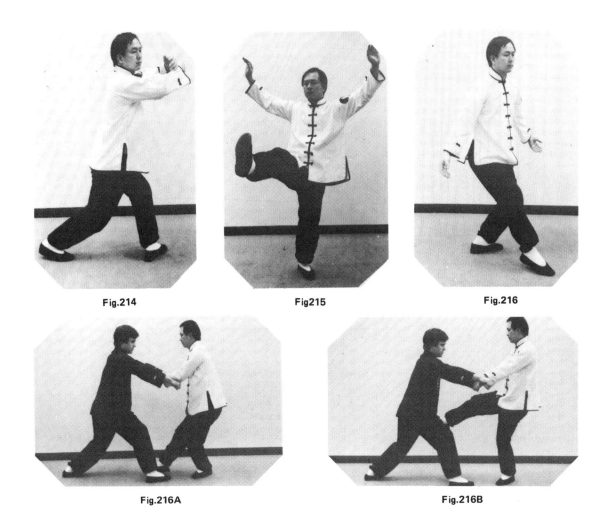

Fig.214   Fig215   Fig.216

Fig.216A   Fig.216B

55. Kick Right (Yu Ti Chiao)

Figure 214: (SW) Turn the upper body to SW while raising your body up to Dsao Pan Bu, crossing your hands. Inhale.

Figure 215: (SW) Repeat 208. Exhale.

56. Attack the Ears by Fists (Shuang Peng Kuan Erg)

Figure 216: (SW) Set the right foot down on its toes and swing your arms down past the right knee. Inhale.

Figure 216A: The defender slides two low punches away.

Figure 216B: The defender then may kick his attacker.

Figure 217: (SW) Both fists swing back, up and in. Exhale.

Figure 217A: After blocking 216A, the defender swings both fists up to attack the opponent's temple.

57. Kick Left (Tso Ti Chiao)

Figure 218: (S) Raise the right knee then step down into Dsao Pan Bu while crossing your arms. Face S. Exhale.

Figure 219: (S) Open both arms and kick with the left heel. Exhale.

Figure 219A: The defender blocks high, then kicks low.

58. Turn and Kick with Heel (270 degrees) (Chuan Shen Teng Chiao)

Figure 220: (W) Bring the left leg in, knee raised and cross your hands. Spin on the right heel 270 degrees counterclockwise. Start to inhale.

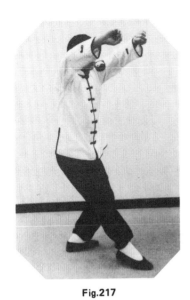

Fig.217

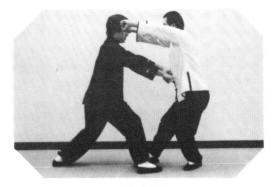

Fig.217A

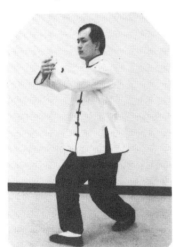

Fig.218

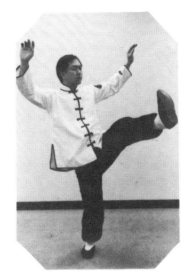

Fig.219

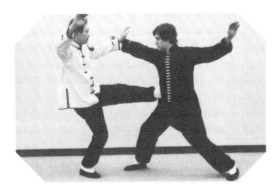

Fig.219A

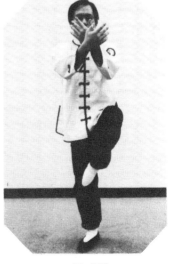

Fig.220

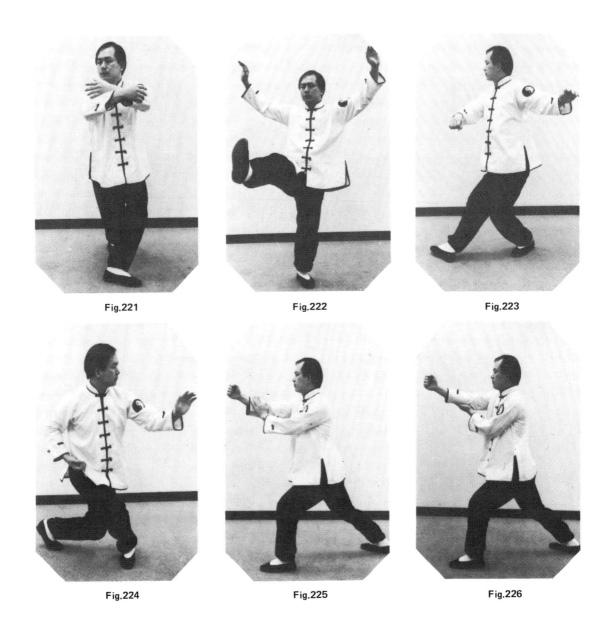

Fig.221   Fig.222   Fig.223

Fig.224   Fig.225   Fig.226

Figure 221: (W) Step the left leg down into Dsao Pan Bu. Complete inhalation.

Figure 222: (W) Repeat 208. Exhale and yell "ha."

59. Twist the Body and Circle Hands (Pieh Shen Ch'ui)

Figure 223: (W) Step the right leg down into Dsao Pan Bu while swinging the right fist down across your body, then up across your body. Start inhalation.

60. Step Forward, Deflect Downward, Parry, and Punch (Chin Pu Pan Lan Ch'ui)

Figures 224 (W), 225 (W). Repeat No. 19.

61. Seal Tightly (Ju Feng Ssu Pi)

Figures 226 (W), 227 (W), 228 (W), 229 (W), 230 (W), and 231 (N). Repeat No. 20.

62. Embrace Tiger and Return to the Mountain (Pao Hu Guei Shan)

Figures 232 (N) and 233 (N). Repeat No. 21.

63. Close Tai Chi (Ho T'ai-Chi)

Figure 234 (N). Repeat No. 22.

84

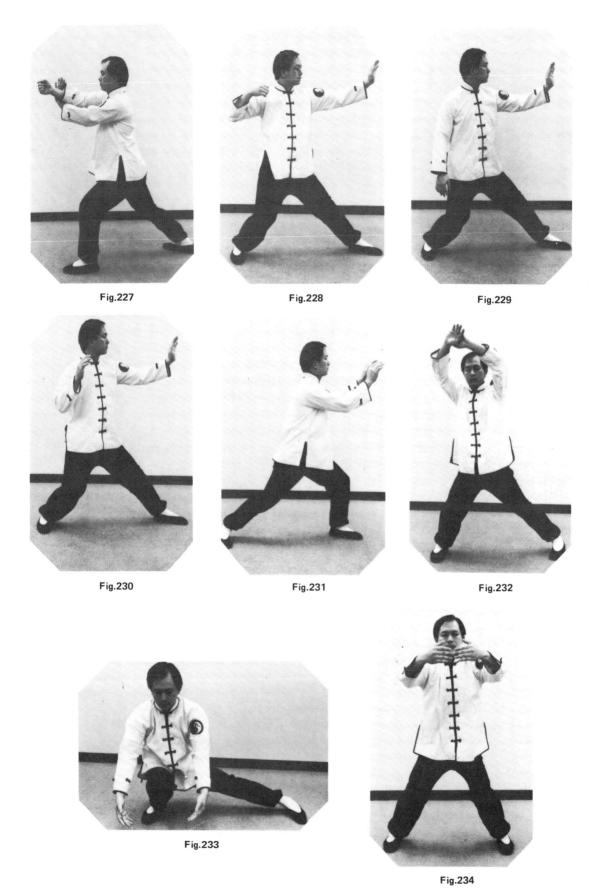

Fig.227

Fig.228

Fig.229

Fig.230

Fig.231

Fig.232

Fig.233

Fig.234

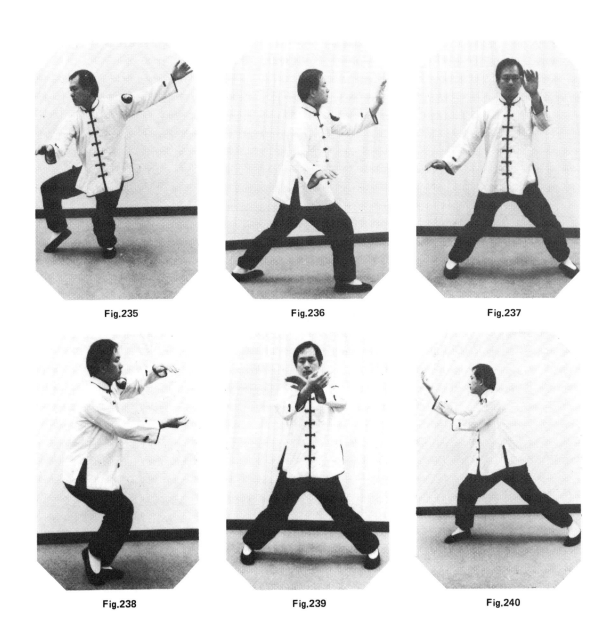

Fig.235 Fig.236 Fig.237

Fig.238 Fig.239 Fig.240

64. Ward-Off, Rollback, Press, and Push (Peng, Lu, Ghi, An)
Figures 235 (E), 236 (E), 237 (N), 238 (W), 239 (N), 240 (E), 241 (E), 242 (E), 243 (E), 244 (E), 245 (E), 246 (E), and 247 (E). Repeat Nos. 4, 5, 6, and 7.

65. Single Whip (Tan Pien)
Figures 248 (N), 249 (W), 250 (W), 251 (W), and 252 (W). Repeat No. 8.

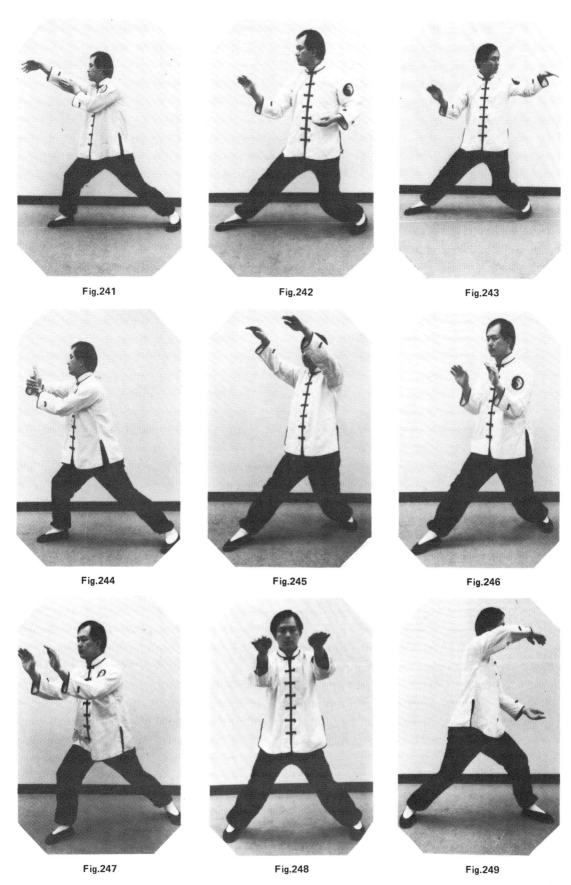

Fig.241 Fig.242 Fig.243

Fig.244 Fig.245 Fig.246

Fig.247 Fig.248 Fig.249

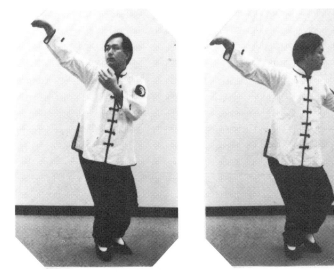

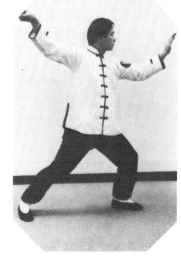

Fig.250   Fig.251   Fig.252

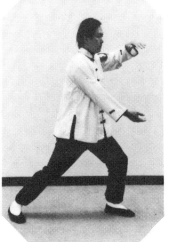

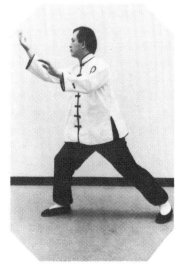

Fig.253   Fig.254

66. Wild Horses Share Mane: Right (Yu Yeh Ma Fen Tsung)
Figure 253: (W) Swing the right hand down and up to the waist height. Inhale.
Figure 254: (E) Turn the body on your heels 180 degrees clockwise while sliding the right hand up. The stance is Deng San Bu. Exhale.
Figure 254A: The defender strikes his opponent's chest.

67. Wild Horses Share Mane: Left (Tso Yeh Ma Fen Tsung)
Figure 255: (NW) Bring the left foot up to the right leg and turn your palms in to face each other, left palm up, right palm down. Inhale.
Figure 256: (NW) Step forward to NW with the left leg into Deng San Bu and slide the left hand up, palm facing in. Breathe out.
Figure 256-A: The defender grabs his opponent's arm with his right hand and strikes up with his left.

68. Wild Horses Share Mane: Right (Yu Yeh Ma Fen Tsung)
Figure 257: (E) Bring the right leg up to the left leg. Turn your palms toward each other, left palm facing down, right palm facing up. Inhale.
Figure 258: (W) Step straight back with the right leg. Turn 180 degrees clockwise while sliding the right hand up, palm facing in. The stance is Deng San Bu. Exhale.

69. Grasp Sparrow's Tail: Left (Tso Lan Ch'iao Wei)
Figure 259: (N) Turn the right palm down, left palm up, and shift N into Ma Bu. Inhale.

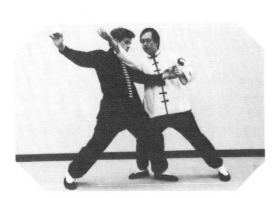

Fig.254A

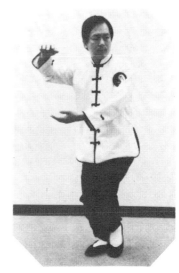

Fig.255

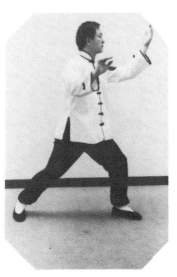

Fig.256

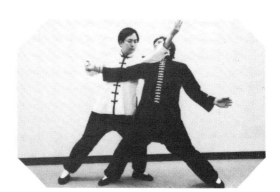

Fig.256A

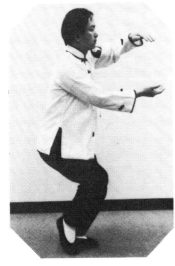

Fig.257

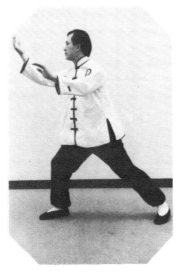

Fig.258

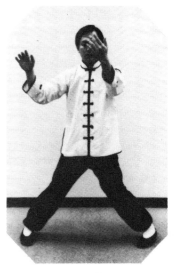

Fig.259

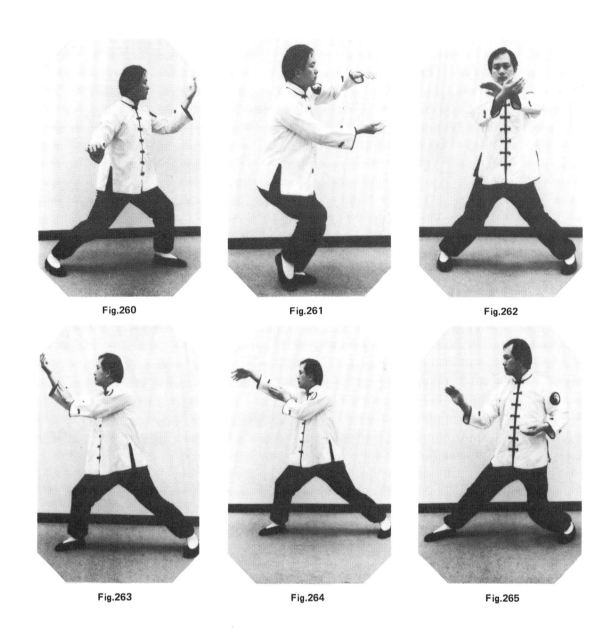

Fig.260   Fig.261   Fig.262

Fig.263   Fig.264   Fig.265

Figure 260: (W) Turn and repeat 59. Exhale.

70. Ward-Off, Rollback, Press, and Push (Peng, Lu, Ghi, An)
Figures 261 (W), 262 (N), 263 (E), 264 (E), 265 (E), 266 (E), 267 (E), 268 (E), 269 (E), and 270 (E). Repeat Nos. 4, 5, 6, and 7.

71. Single Whip (Tan Pien)
Figures 271 (N), 272 (N), 273 (W), 274 (W), and 275 (W). Repeat No. 8.

90

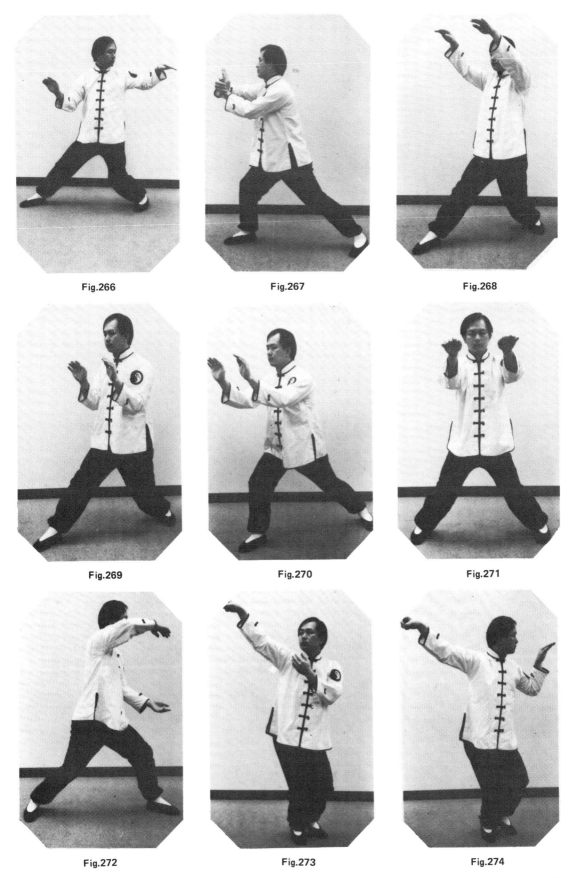

Fig.266   Fig.267   Fig.268

Fig.269   Fig.270   Fig.271

Fig.272   Fig.273   Fig.274

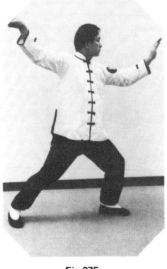

Fig.275

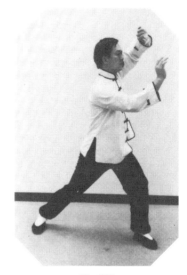

Fig.276

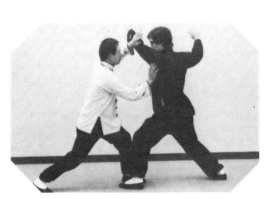

Fig.276A

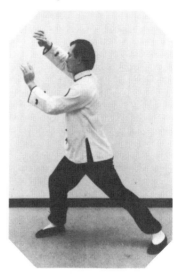

Fig.277

72. Fair Lady Weaves Shuttle: Left (Tso Yu Nu Ch'uan Suo)

Figure 276: (W) Lower both arms to waist level. Breathe in. Raise the left arm up and push the right palm forward. Breathe out.

Figure 276A: As the opponent attacks, the defender pushes his power up and attacks his opponent's side.

73. Fair Lady Weaves Shuttle: Right (Yu Yu Nu Ch'uan Suo)

Figure 277: (E) Turn 180 degrees clockwise on your heels while lowering both arms to waist level. Breathe in. Shift the stance into Deng San Bu and raise the right hand while pushing the left palm forward. Breathe out.

Figure 277A: Same as 276A except the hands are switched.

74. Fair Lady Weaves Shuttle: Left (Tso Yu Nu Ch'uan Suo)

Figure 278: (SW) Bring the left leg up to the right leg. Begin to breathe in.

Figure 279: (SW) Step the left leg back to SW. Lower both arms to waist level and begin to turn 135 degrees counterclockwise on your heels. Finish inhalation. Complete the turn; stance is Deng San Bu, while raising the left arm and pushing the right palm out. Breathe out.

75. Fair Lady Weaves Shuttle: Right (Yu Yu Nu Ch'uan Suo)

Figure 280: (SW) Bring the right leg to the left leg. Begin to breathe in.

Figure 281 (E) Step straight back with the right leg and lower your hands to waist level while turning 180 degrees clockwise on your heels. Breathe in. Shift into Deng San Bu and raise your right arm while pushing the left palm out. Exhale.

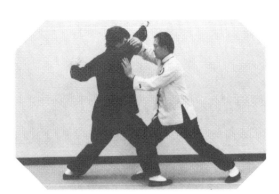

Fig.277A

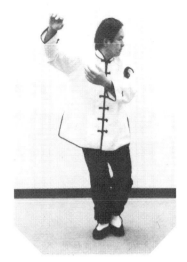

Fig.278

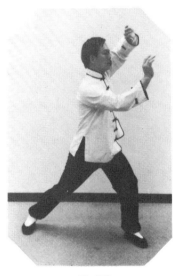

Fig.279

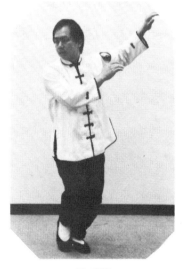

Fig.280

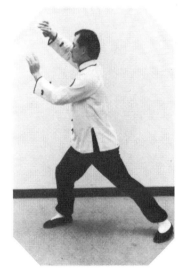

Fig.281

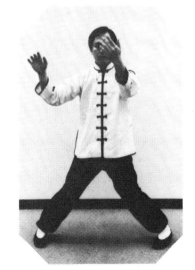

Fig.282

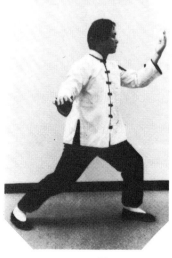

Fig.283

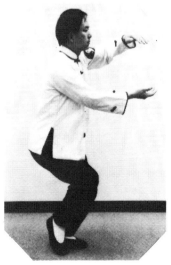

Fig.284

93

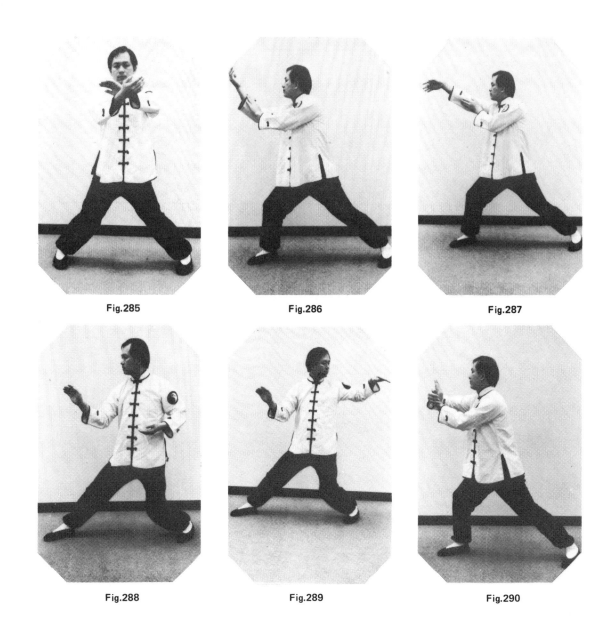

Fig.285   Fig.286   Fig.287

Fig.288   Fig.289   Fig.290

76. Grasp Sparrow's Tail: Left (Tso Lan Ch'iao Wei)

Figure 282: (N) Turn the right palm up and repeat 58. Inhale.

Figure 283: (W) Repeat 59. Exhale.

77. Ward-Off, Rollback, Press and Push (Peng, Lu, Ghi, An)

Figure 284 (W), 285 (N), 286 (E), 287 (E), 288 (E), 289 (E), 290 (E), 291 (E), 292 (E) and 293 (E).
   Repeat Nos. 4, 5, 6, and 7.

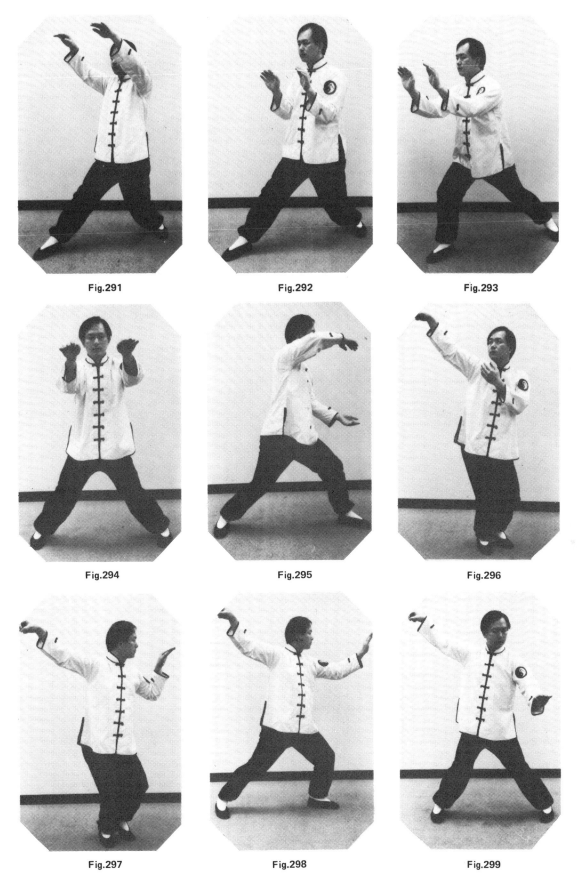

Fig.291   Fig.292   Fig.293

Fig.294   Fig.295   Fig.296

Fig.297   Fig.298   Fig.299

95

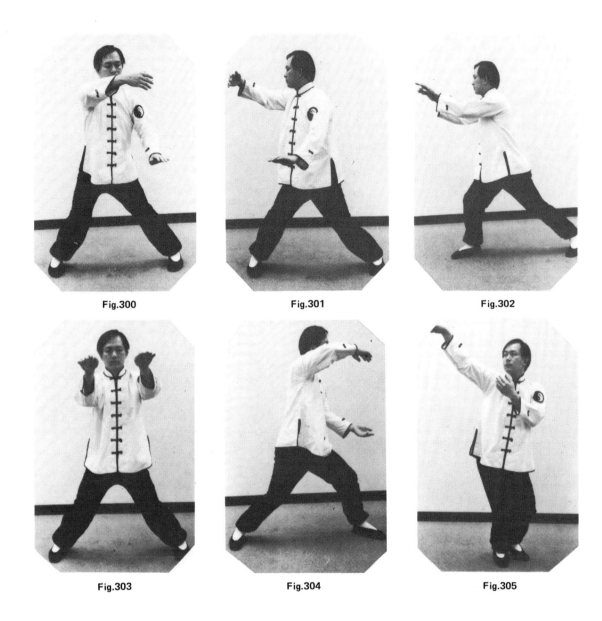

Fig.300 Fig.301 Fig.302

Fig.303 Fig.304 Fig.305

78. **Single Whip (Tan Pien)**
Figures 294 (N), 295 (W), 296 (W), 297 (W), and 298 (W). Repeat No. 8.

79. **Wave Hands in Clouds: Right (Yu Yun Shou)**
Figures 299 (N), 300 (N), 301 (N), and 302 (E). Repeat No. 39.

80. **Single Whip (Tan Pien)**
Figurs 303 (N), 304 (W), 305 (W), and 307 (W). Repeat No. 8.

81. **Lower the Snake Body (Shih Shen Hsia Shih)**
Figure 308: (W) Sit back in Ssu Lieu Bu and move the left arm back. Begin to breathe in.
Figure 309: (W) Squat into Fu Hu Bu, weight on the right leg. Swing the left hand past your face and down to the left foot. Complete inhalation.
Figure 309A: The defender slides the punch away while squatting down.
Figure 309B: While squatting, the defender slides away from the opponent's kick.

82. **Golden Rooster Stands By One Leg: Right (Yu Chin Chi Tu Li)**
Figure 310: (W) Shift your weight forward into Deng San Bu, the left leg forward, while moving the right hand down and up. Begin to exhale.

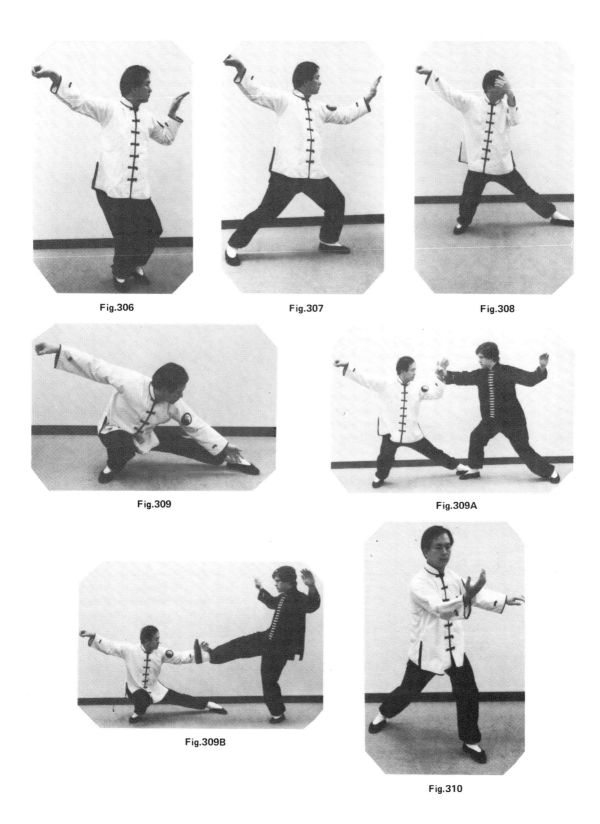

Fig.306

Fig.307

Fig.308

Fig.309

Fig.309A

Fig.309B

Fig.310

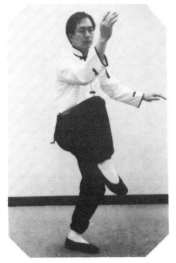

Fig.311

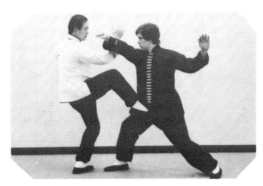

Fig.311A

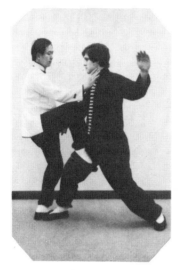

Fig.311B

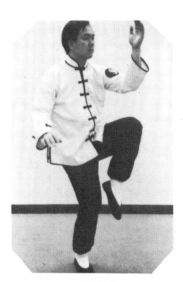

Fig.312

Figure 311: (W) Bring the right leg up while moving the right hand to face height, turning the palm to the side. Complete exhalation.

Figure 311A: The defender simultaneously blocks and kicks the opponent.

Figure 311B: The defender may use his right hand to grab the throat.

83 Golden Rooster Stands By One Leg: Left (Tso Chin Chi Tu Li)

Figure 312: (W) Step down with the right leg and lower the right hand, palm down to waist level. Breathe in. Raise the left knee and hand, palm facing to the side. Breathe out.

Figure 312A: The defender slides the punch away on the inside and kicks the groin.

84. Step Back and Repulse Monkey: Left (Tso Tao Nien Hou)

Figures 313 (W), 314 (W), and 315 (W). Repeat No. 26.

85. Diagonal Flying (Hsieh Fei Shih)

Figures 316 (S), and 317 (N). Repeat No. 29.

96. Lift Hands and Lean Forward (T'i Shou Shang Shih)

Figures 318 (N), and 319 (N). Repeat No. 9.

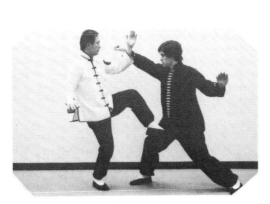

Fig.312A

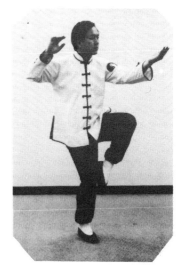

Fig.313

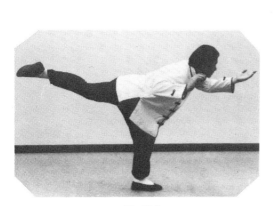

Fig.314

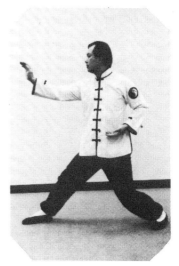

Fig.315

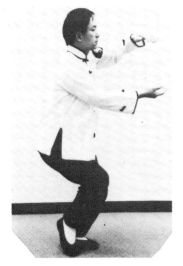

Fig.316

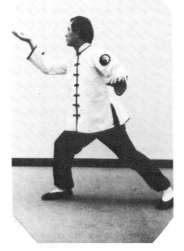

Fig.317

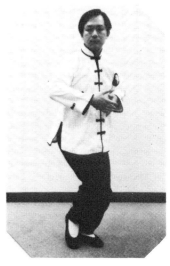

Fig.318

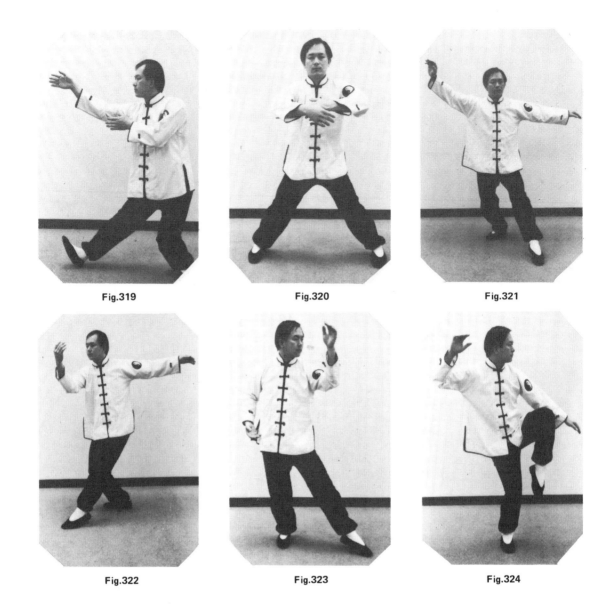

Fig.319　　　　　　Fig.320　　　　　　Fig.321

Fig.322　　　　　　Fig.323　　　　　　Fig.324

87. Crane Spreads Its Wings (Pai Hao Liang Ch'ih)
　　Figures 320 (N), and 321 (W). Repeat No. 10.
88. Brush Knee and Step Forward: Left (Tso Lou Hsi Yao Pu)
　　Figures 322 (N), 323 (W), 324 (W), and 325 (W). Repeat No. 11.
89. Pick Up the Needle From the Sea Bottom (Hai Ti Lao Chen)
　　Figures 326 (W), and 327 (W). Repeat No. 33.
90. Fan Back (Shan T'ung Pei)
　　Figures 328 (W), and 329 (W). Repeat No. 34.
91　White Snake Turns Body and Spits Poison (Chuan Shen Pai She T'u Hsin)
　　Figure 330: (E) Turn the upper body to E while sitting back in Ssu Lieu Bu and sweeping the right
　　　　hand down. Inhale.
　　Figure 331: (E) Swing the right hand to the side. Shift the stance forward into Deng San Bu and push
　　　　with the left palm. Exhale.
　　Figure 331A: The defender sweeps a low punch away and attacks his opponent's chest.

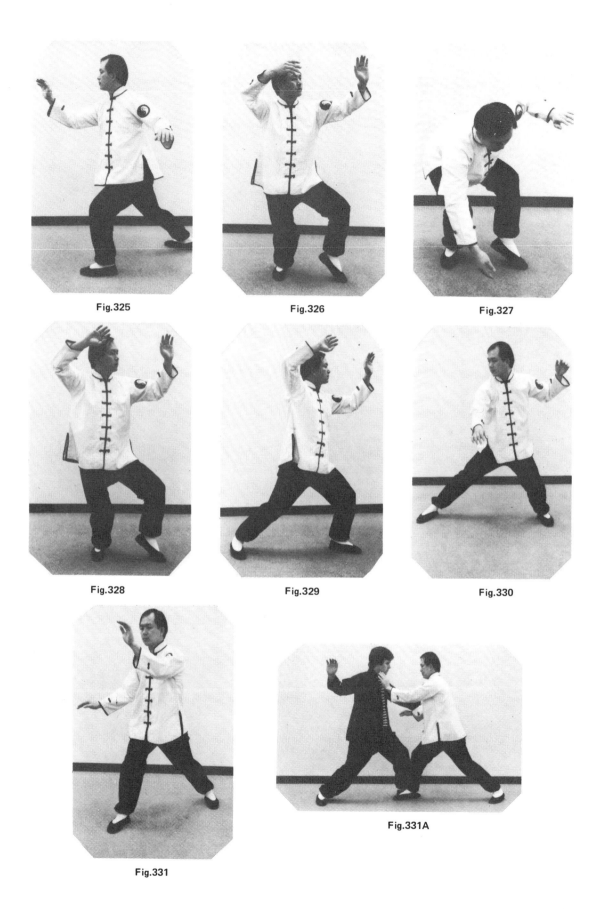

Fig.325

Fig.326

Fig.327

Fig.328

Fig.329

Fig.330

Fig.331

Fig.331A

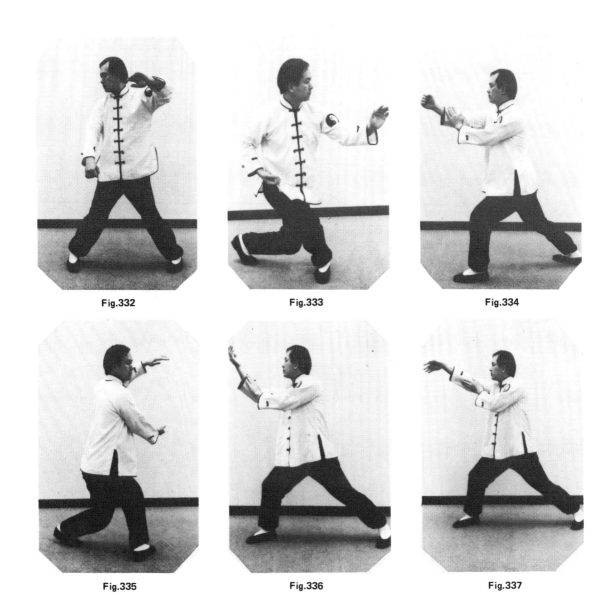

Fig.332   Fig.333   Fig.334

Fig.335   Fig.336   Fig.337

92. **Step Forward, Deflect Downward, Parry, and Punch (Chin Pu Pan Lan Ch'ui)**
 Figures 332 (E), 333 (E), and 334 (E). Repeat No. 36.
93. **Step Forward, Ward-Off, Rollback, Press, and Push (Shang Pu Peng, Lu, Ghi, An)**
 Figures 335 (E), 336 (E), 337 (E), 338 (E), 339 (E), 340 (E), 341 (E), 342 (E), and 343 (E). Repeat
 No. 37.
94. **Single Whip (Tan Pien)**
 Figures 344 (N), 345 (N), 346 (N), 347 (W), and 348 (W). Repeat No. 8.

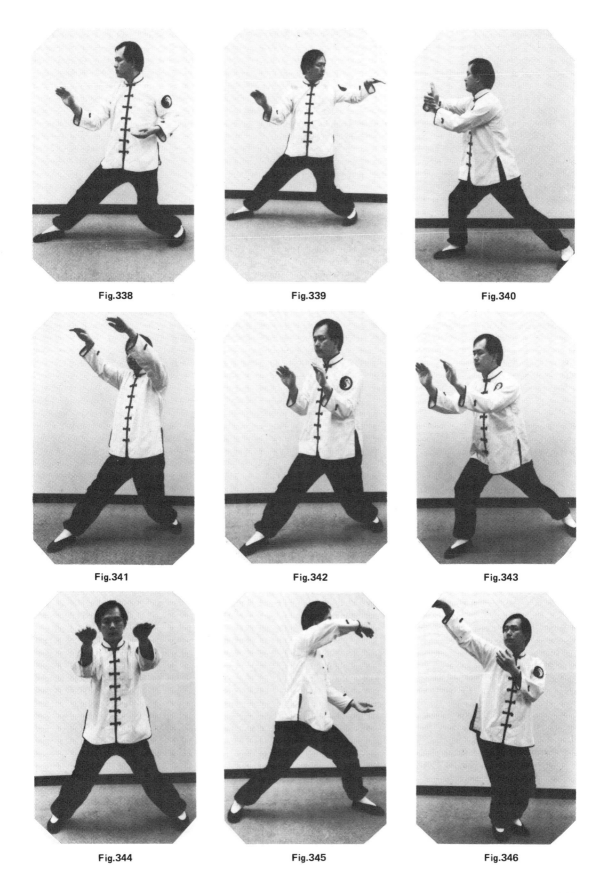

Fig.338

Fig.339

Fig.340

Fig.341

Fig.342

Fig.343

Fig.344

Fig.345

Fig.346

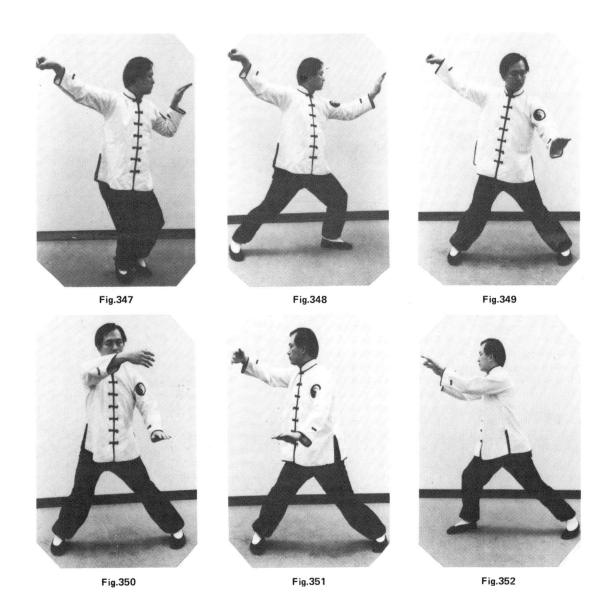

Fig.347   Fig.348   Fig.349

Fig.350   Fig.351   Fig.352

95. Wave Hands in Clouds: Right (Yu Yun Sou)
   Figures 349 (N), 350 (N), and 351 (E). Repeat No. 39.
96. Single Whip (Tan Pien)
   Figures 352 (E), 353 (N), 354 (N), 355 (W), 356 (W), and 357 (W). Repeat No. 8.
97. Stand High to Search Out the Horse (Kao T'an Ma)
   Figure 358 (W). Repeat No. 43.
98. Cross Hands (Shih Tzu Shou)
   Figure 359: (W) Shift into Deng San Bu. Swing the right forearm down across the body. The left arm
      is inside the right. Move the right hand under the left elbow and turn the left palm in. Exhale.
      Similar in use to 134A.
99. Turn and Kick (Chuan Shen Shih Tzu T'ui)
   Figure 360: (E) Turn 180 degrees clockwise while shifting the weight onto your left leg; the right
      foot is on its toes. Cross your hands and inhale.

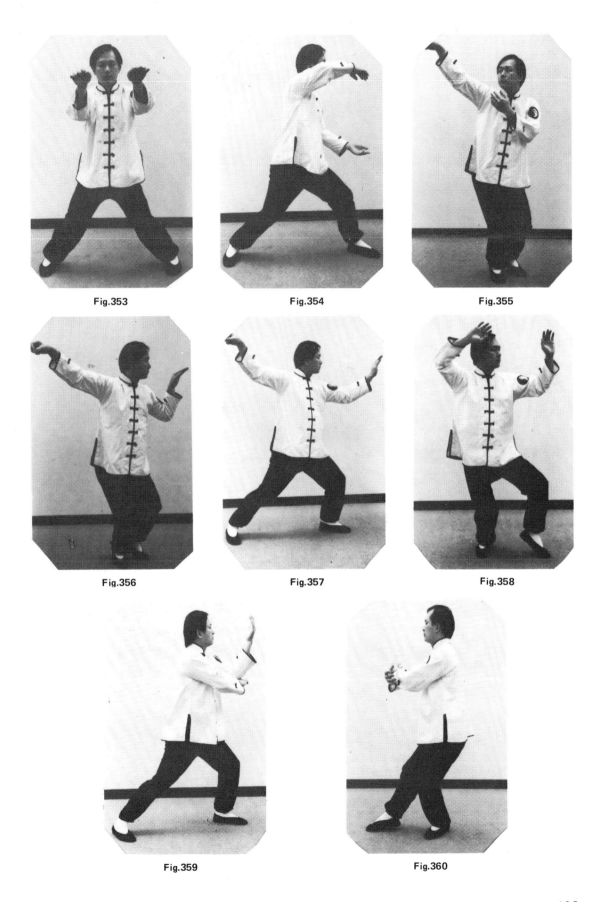

Fig.353

Fig.354

Fig.355

Fig.356

Fig.357

Fig.358

Fig.359

Fig.360

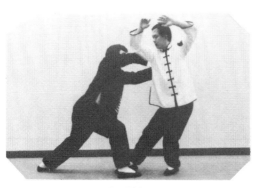

Fig.360A

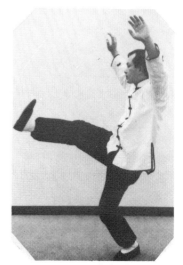

Fig.361

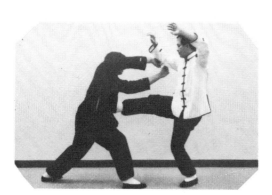

Fig.361A

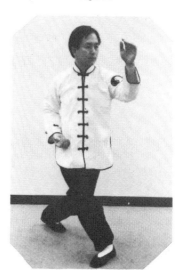

Fig. 362

Figure 360A: The defender turns as he is grabbed from the rear.

Figure 361: (E) Spread your arms open and kick with the right heel. Exhale.

Figure 361A: The defender kicks the opponent after turning.

100. Brush Knee and Punch Down (Lou Hsi Chih Tang Ch'ui)

Figure 362: (E) Step down with the right leg into Dsao Pan Bu and swing the left arm down across the body. Withdraw the right fist to the waist. Inhale.

Figure 363: (E) Step forward with the left leg into Deng San Bu and punch down with the right fist. Exhale.

Figure 363A: The defender sweeps a punch away and attacks the muscle above the knee.

101. Step Forward, Ward-Off, Rollback, Press, and Push (Shang Pu P'eng, Lu, Ghi, An)

Figures 364 (E), 365 (E), 366 (E), 367 (E), 368 (E), 369 (E), 370 (E), 371 (E), and 372 (E). Repeat Nos. 4, 5, 6, and 7.

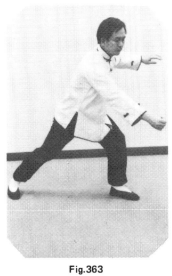

Fig.363

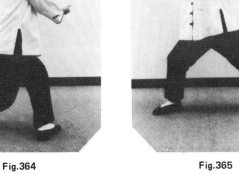

Fig.363A

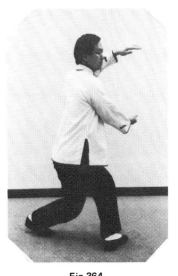

Fig.364

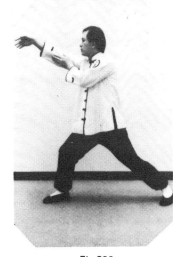

Fig.365

Fig.366

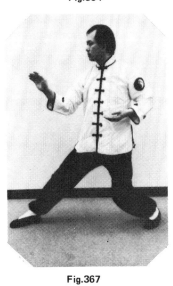

Fig.367

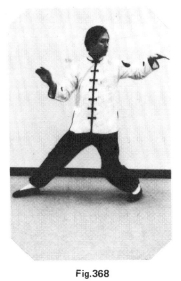

Fig.368

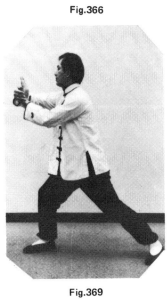

Fig.369

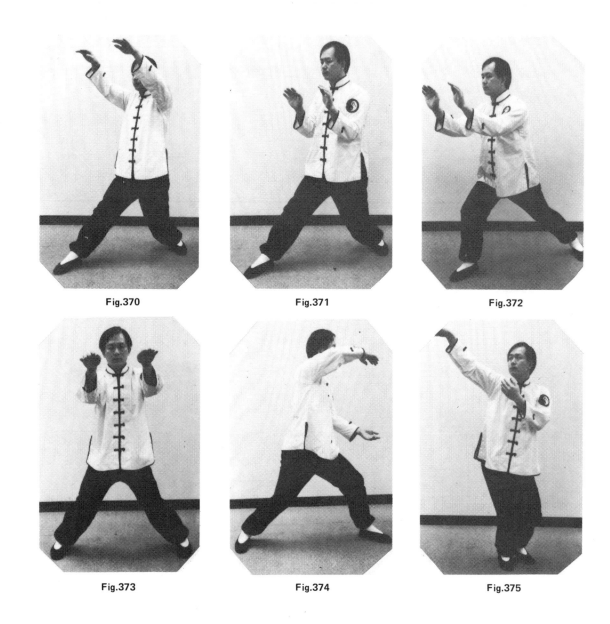

Fig.370   Fig.371   Fig.372

Fig.373   Fig.374   Fig.375

102. Single Whip (Tan Pien)
Figures 373 (N), 374 (N) 375 (W), 376 (W), and 377 (W). Repeat No. 8.

103. Lower the Snake Body (Shih Shen Hsia Shih)
Figures 378 (W) and 379 (W). Repeat No. 81.

104. Step Forward to Seven Stars (Shang Pu Ch'i Hsing)
Figure 380: (W) Raise the body up and lift the left fist up. Step the right foot forward on its toes.
    Punch with the right fist under the left hand. Exhale.
Figure 380A: The defender blocks with the left hand, then punches to his opponent's armpit.
Figure 380B: The defender may also block from the inside position and then kick.

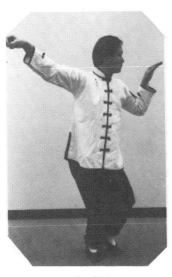

Fig.376

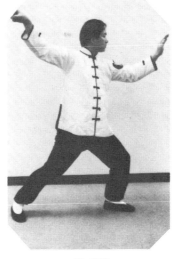

Fig.377

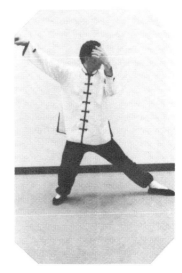

Fig.378

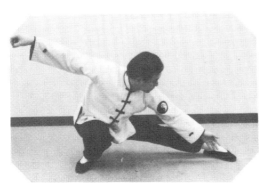

Fig.379

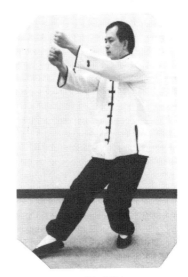

Fig.380

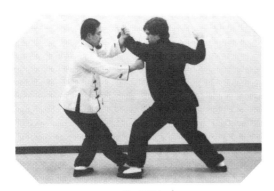

Fig.380A

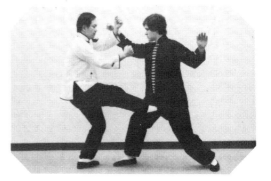

Fig.380B

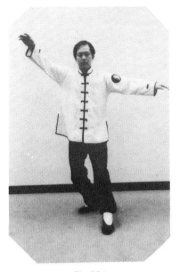

Fig.381

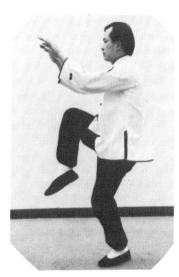

Fig.381A

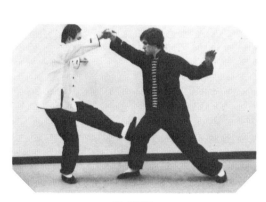

Fig.381B

Fig.382

105. Step Back and Ride the Tiger (T'ui Pu K'ua Fu)

Figure 381: (W) Step back with the right leg. Raise the left foot on its toes, and spread your arms. Move your right palm forward. Inhale.

Figure 381A: The defender blocks a high punch.

Figure 381B: The defender may kick the knee.

106. Turn Body and Sweep Lotus with Leg. (Chuan Shen Pai Lien)

Figure 382: (W) Raise the right knee up. Move the hands down, palms up. Slide both hands up, crossing then uncrossing them, while turning the palms down. Exhale.

Figure 382A: The opponent grabs the defender; the defender slides his hands up to the attacker's eyes and kicks the groin.

Figures 383: (W) Swing the right leg behind and across the left leg. Breathe in.

Figure 383A: The attacker grabs the defender's back. By stepping the right leg back and across, the defender can turn his body to dissolve the hold.

Figure 383B: The defender turns around and grabs his opponent's hair. The defender may pull the opponent down.

Figure 384: (E) Turn your body 180 degrees on its heels to face E; the stance is Ma Bu. Sweep the right leg in a clockwise circle. Slap both hands with your leg at the top of the circle. Exhale.

Figure 384A: After turning his body, the defender sweeps and hits the opponent's back.

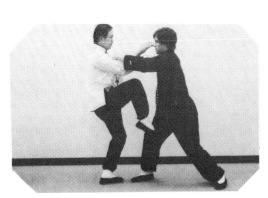

Fig.382A

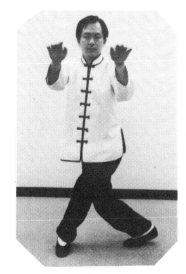

Fig.383

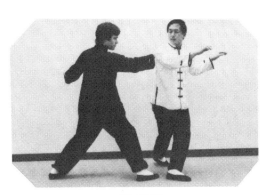

Fig.383A

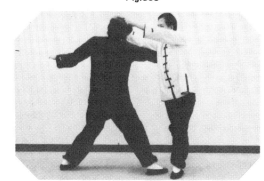

Fig.383B

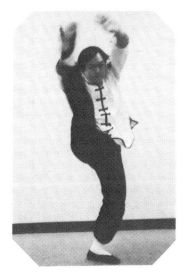

Fig.384

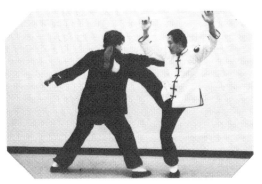

Fig.384A

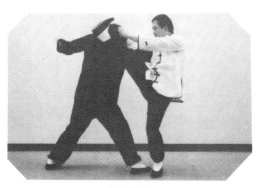

Fig.384B

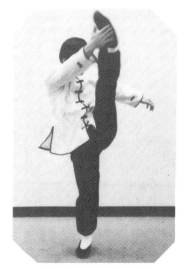

Fig.385

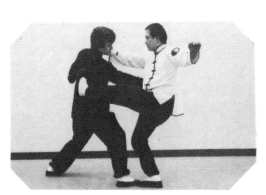

Fig.385A

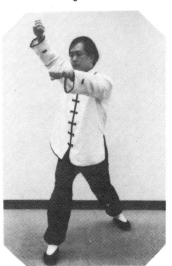

Fig.386

Figure 384B: If the defender grabs the opponent's hair, he pushes his opponent's head into the kick.

Figure 385: (E) Set the right leg down. Sweep the left leg out, up and then in; the heel is flat when the hand slaps it at the highest point. Inhale and exhale.

Figure 385A: The defender may also kick the side of the opponent's body while pushing in.

107. Draw the Bow and Shoot the Tiger (Wan Kung She Fu)

Figure 386: (W) Place your left foot to the rear, move the right fist up, and punch the left fist forward. The stance is Deng San Bu. Inhale and Exhale.

Figure 386A: The defender deflects the punch up and attacks his opponent's chest.

108. Twist Body and Circle Hand (Pieh Shen Ch'ui)

Figure 387: (W) Make a clockwise circle with the right arm in front of the body. Begin to inhale.

109. Step Forward, Deflect Downward, Parry, and Punch (Chin Pu Pan Lan Ch'ui)

Figures 388 (W), and 389 (W). Repeat No. 19.

110. Seal Tightly (Ju Feng Ssu Pi)

Figures 390 (W), 391 (W), 392 (W), 393 (W), 394 (W), and 395 (W). Repeat No. 20.

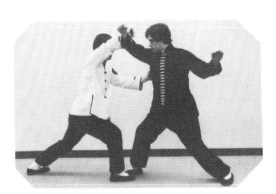

Fig.386A

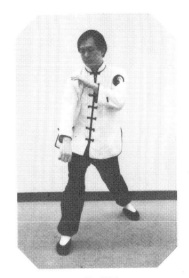

Fig.387

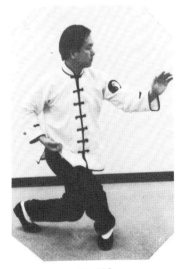

Fig.388

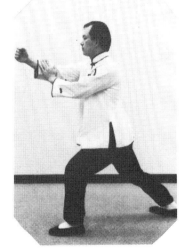

Fig.389

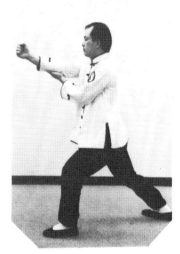

Fig.390

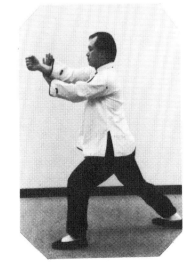

Fig.391

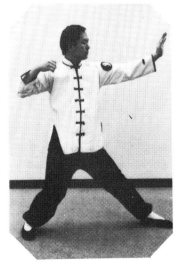

Fig.392

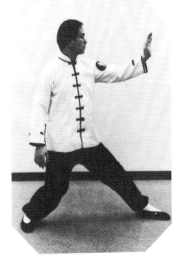

Fig.393

113

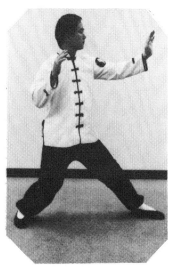

Fig.394

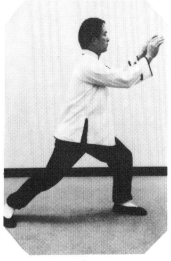

Fig.395

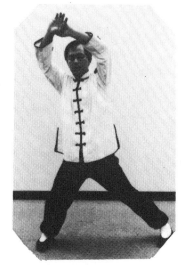

Fig.396

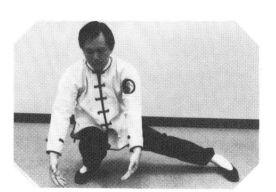

Fig.397

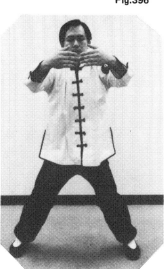

Fig.398

111. Embrace the Tiger and Return to the Mountain (Pao Hu Guei Shan)
　　Figures 396 (N), and 397 (N). Repeat No. 21.
112. Close Tai Chi (Ho Tai-Chi)
　　Figure 398 (N). Repeat No. 22.
　　Figure 399 (N) Extend your arms, palms down, and raise the left knee. Begin to inhale.
113. Return to the Original Stance (T'ai-Chi Huan Yuan)
　　Figure 400: (N) Step back with the left leg. Finish inhalation.
　　Figure 400A: (N) Step back with the right leg. Finish inhalation.
　　Figure 401: (N) Lower the arms so the original stance is assumed. Complete exhalation.

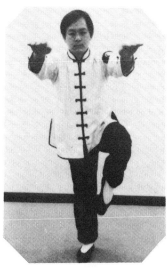

Fig.399

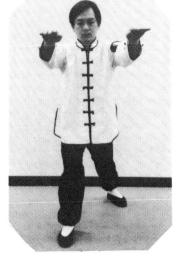

Fig.400

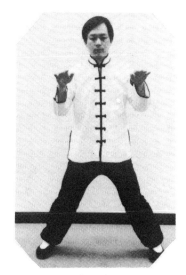

Fig.400A

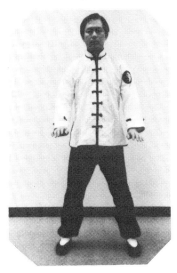

Fig.401

Pushing Hands

Pushing hands is the foundation of Tai Chi free fighting. When the student first starts these drills, he and his partner should do the forms slowly while coordinating the technique with breathing; inhale while defending, and exhale while attacking. In all, the student should follow all the rules for breathing that were stated in this chapter and Chapter 2. Later, when the practitioners become more proficient, they can increase the speed and power.

Basically, there are five major aspects of fighting which are trained during pushing hands. First, by pushing hands the practitioner learns how to "listen" to his opponent's power. This is why the techniques are done very slowly at first; the practitioner must build up the sensitivity of his skin to the opponent's movements. Second, pushing hands develops the ability to stick or adhere to an opponent. By constant practice, the Tai Chi martial artist will learn how to follow the other's power with ease.

Third, pushing hands trains the generation of internal power by the constant application of the three vectors for power; the rear leg is mentally pushed back, the chi is pushed down while expanding the Dan Tien, and the striking arm is pushed forward. Fourth, because any fighting must be dynamic, pushing hands will, in some techniques, train the legs to move with stability and smoothness. Finally, by practicing pushing hands, the Tai Chi martial artist gains invaluable experience.

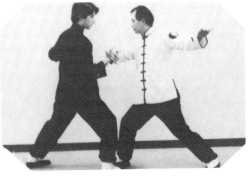

Fig.402

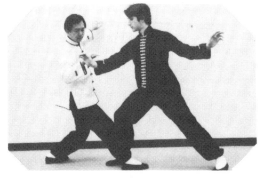

Fig.403

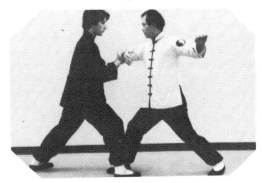

Fig.404

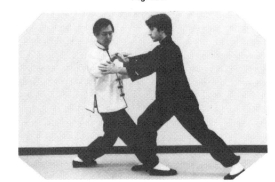

Fig.405

Technique 1

Figure 402: B (person in black top) pushes W's (person in white top) wrist.

Figure 403: W turns his waist and arms to the right to guide B's power to the side. W then pushes toward B's chest, keeping contact with or sticking on B's hand. B then turns his waist and right arm to the right to dissolve W's power. B attacks again.

Technique 2

Figure 404: B pushes W' right arm with both hands.

Figure 405: W turns his waist and arm to the right side, dissolving B's power.

Figure 406: As W guides B's power to the side, W's left hand assists by sliding B's elbow also to the side. W then pushes B with both hands. B resolves the push the same way as W did.

Technique 3

Figure 407: B pushes as in figure 404 To resolve B's power, W turns his right arm and waist to the left.

Figure 408: At the same time that W turns to the left, W slides his left hand under B's left hand.

Figure 409: By using his left hand, W slides away both of B's hands to the left. W then pushes while sticking to B's left arm. B resolves by turning his body to the right. Next, B slides away both of W's hands in order to push. Techniques 2 and 3 may be done together.

Technique 4

Figure 410: Practitioners stand with opposite legs forward. B pushed at W's chest. W guides the power down by covering B's arm.

Figure 411: W then pushes at B's chest. B moves his hand up to guide W's power to the side. B then pushes, with W either guiding the power down, or by sliding his hand around B's wrist so the power is resolved up to the side. In the last method, W's hand will finally be in the same position as B's. B may counter by using either method: guiding the power down or to the side.

Technique 5

Figure 412: This is a two-handed version. Both practitioners stand with the same leg forward. Each of the counters represents an option which the student has on any attack. Therefore, the individuals should try to do the techniques smoothly and spontaneously. In this pushing hands technique, the student flows into any counter move that he wants. B pushes W's chest. W slides the power down.

Figure 413: W pushes up at B's chest. B slides the power up and to the sides.

116

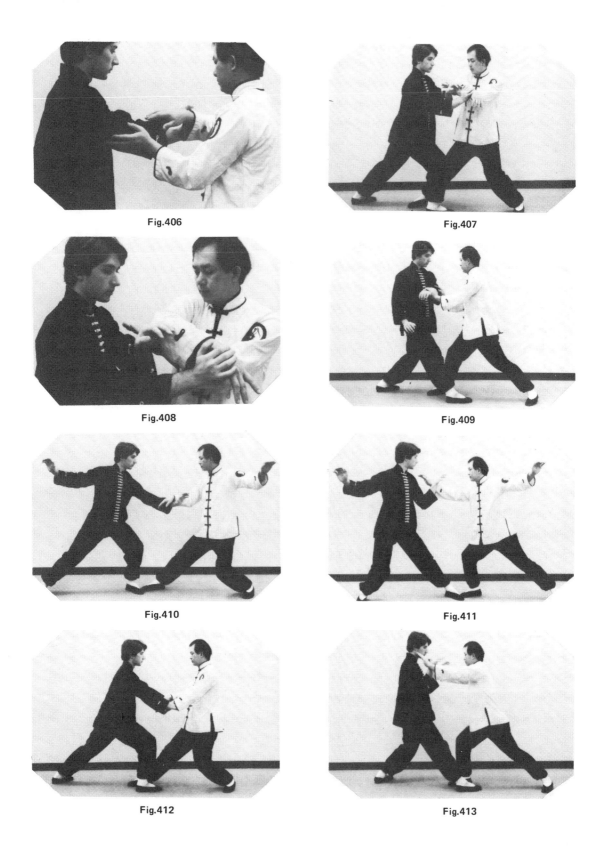

Fig.406

Fig.407

Fig.408

Fig.409

Fig.410

Fig.411

Fig.412

Fig.413

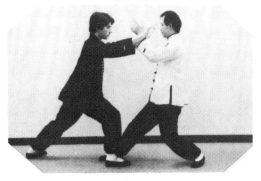

Fig.414

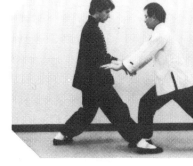

Fig.415

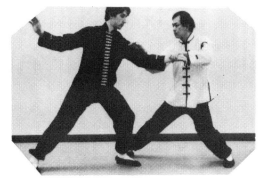

Fig.416

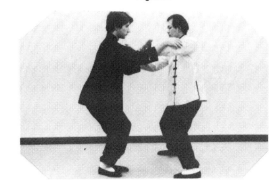

Fig.417

Figure 414: B pushes at W's chest. W slides his hands under B's push and guides the power up.

Figure 415: W pushes at B's chest. B slides the power down.

Technique 6

Figure 416: W grabs B's wrist with his left hand and pulls. At the same time, W places his right arm above B's elbow to exert extra pressure.

Figure 417: To counter, B steps with his right leg along the line of W's pull. As B steps forward, his right arm swings around W's left elbow.

Figure 418: B brings his left leg around so that he is perpendicular to W. B then pulls on W.

Technique 7

Figure 419: B presses on W's chest.

Figure 420: W crosses his left leg behind his body, turns his waist, and slides his left arm up to B's left hand.

Figure 421: W sets himself to B's side and presses.

Figure 422: The next two photographs represent a second option which W can have when he is pressed as in figure 419. As B attempts to press, W slides his right hand across B's arm to guide the attack to the side.

Figure 423: W then lifts his right leg and steps behind B to press him from behind. When the practitioners use this pushing hands exercise, both methods are combined and done in a fluid and spontaneous manner.

Technique 8

Figure 424: W grabs B's arm and steps in to strike B with the forearm. W's leg is set behind B.

Figure 425: To counter, B must quickly pull his own right arm in. As B pulls, he also presses his left hand against W's elbow.

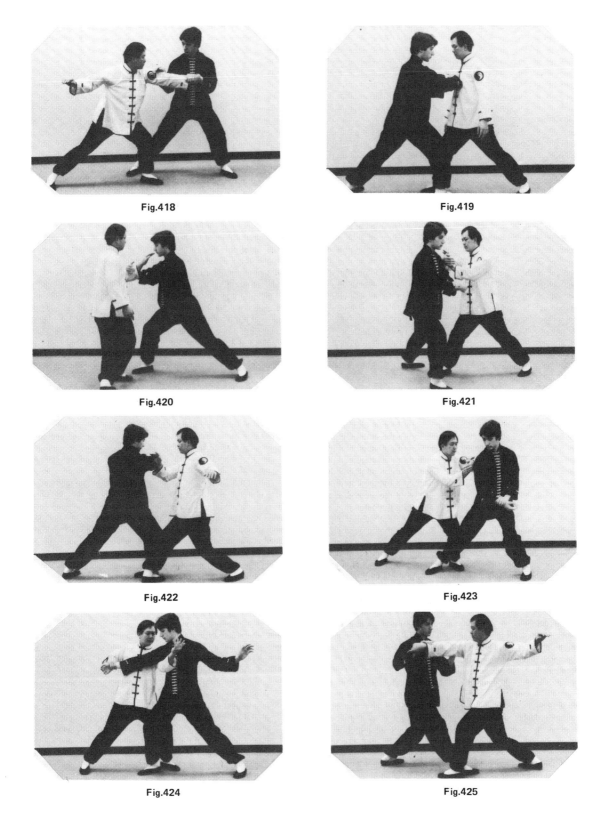

Fig.418

Fig.419

Fig.420

Fig.421

Fig.422

Fig.423

Fig.424

Fig.425

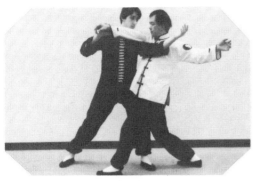

Fig.426

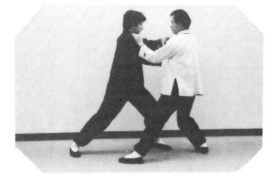

Fig.427

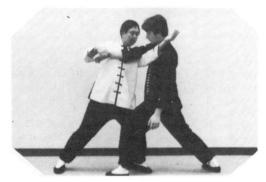

Fig.428

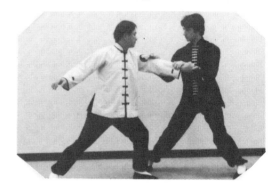

Fig.429

Figure 426: B switches legs and attacks B's chest with his left arm.

Figure 427: W pulls his right arm back along with B's arm.

Figure 428: W then attacks B's chest from underneath. To counter, B pulls, switches legs, and attacks W's chest from underneath.

Technique 9

Figure 429: B pulls on W's left arm.

Figure 430: W brings his left arm back while pushing B's right hand forward. As W pulls his hands away, his left knee is raised.

Figure 431: W steps down behing B and strikes B's head with his left fist.

Figure 432: To counter, B steps back with his right leg and pulls W's arm.

Figure 433: W pulls his right arm back while pushing B's left hand. At the same time, W lifts his right knee.

Figure 434: W steps behind B and strikes the back of B's head. To counter, B steps to the rear with his left leg while pulling on W's right arm.

Technique 10

Figure 435: B punches at W's temple from outside to in with both fists. W slides the power to the side from the inside.

Figure 436: W then punches down with both fists. B slides the power to the outside by moving his hands to an inside position.

Figure 437: B punches with both hands straight down. W slides his hands to the inside and guides B's power to the side.

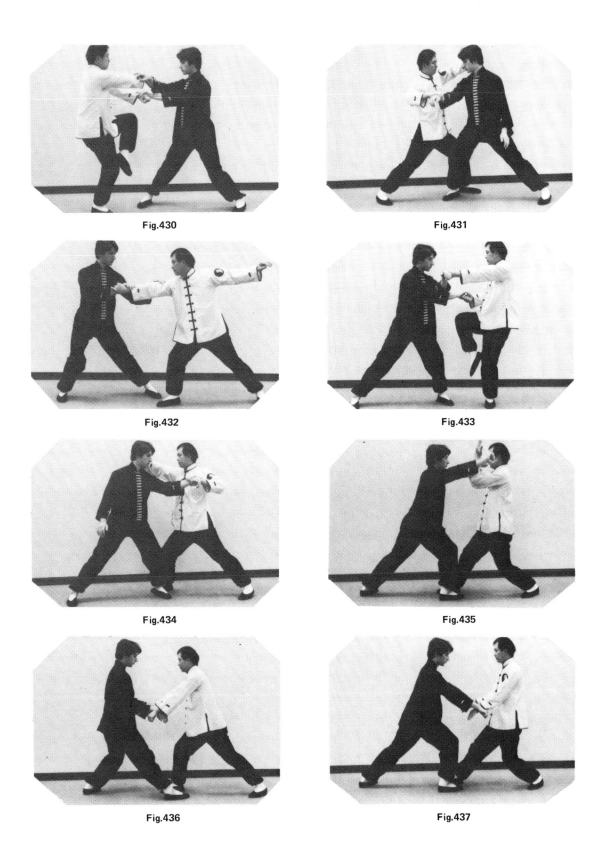

Fig.430

Fig.431

Fig.432

Fig.433

Fig.434

Fig.435

Fig.436

Fig.437

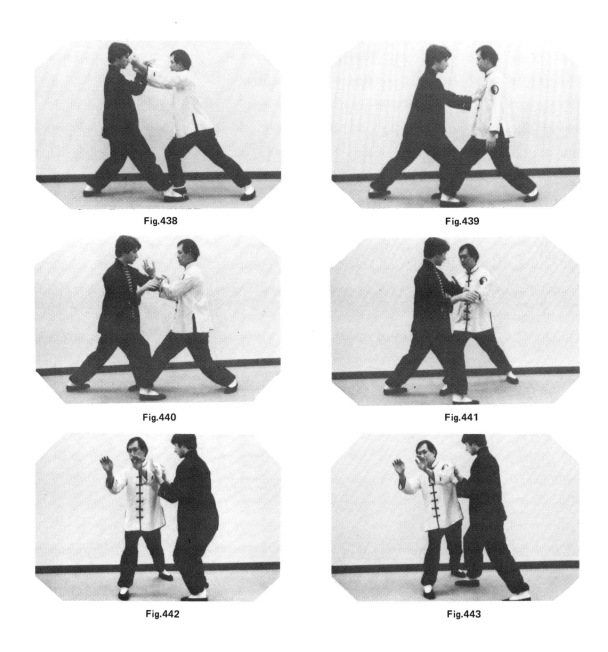

Fig.438

Fig.439

Fig.440

Fig.441

Fig.442

Fig.443

Figure 438: W uppercuts with both fists. B slides his hands from underneath to dissolve the power.

Technique 11

Figure 439: B pushes W's chest.

Figure 440: W slides his left arm under B's arms to guide the push away.

Figure 441: W steps to the side and pushes B with both hands.

Figure 442: B swings his left hand to the side to slide W's push away while also beginning to move laterally.

Figure 443: B sets himself and pushes with both hands. To counter, W slides away from B's push and steps to the side in order to push B.

Tai Chi Barehand Fighting Sequence

The purpose of Tai Chi barehand fighting sequence is to give the student a basis for real fighting by taking techniques from the solo barehand sequence and applying them, in a dynamic fashion, against a real opponent. When the Tai Chi fighting sequence is started, the partners start slowly to insure that the techniques are accurate and the breathing correct; inhalation and exhalation follow the same guidelines as those set down for the solo Tai Chi sequence. Once the form and breathing are correct, the students begin to build up and intensify their practice so that six basic traits will eventually be developed.

The first goal is to develop all those traits which pushing hands trains; adhering, listening, neutralizing, etc. Second, the two-man fighting sequence trains the active application of techniques used for actual fighting. The third trait which the fighting sequence develops is the capacity for unified and dynamic movement, coordinating all parts of the body while the martial artist moves in various directions. Fourth, the martial artist learns how to neutralize his opponent's power while coordinating the technique with a sunken stance: the defender neutralizes his opponent while pushing off his rear leg, lowering his chi, and guiding the waist and hands in the desired direction. Fifth, the students develop the ability to follow each other's speed, thus anticipating any possible movement. Last, the practitioners train their eyes, power, speed, coordination, listening ability, etc., until those traits become second nature.

When the students practice the Tai Chi fighting sequence they should constantly discuss and research the key aspects of various techniques. Every technique contains a movement which is vital for its effective use. Only by actual practice and discussion can these points be discovered. Once the fighting sequence is mastered, the Tai Chi martial artist will have the potential for proficient free fighting.

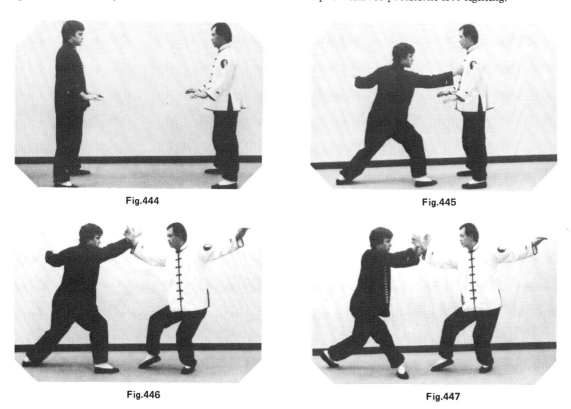

Fig.444

Fig.445

Fig.446

Fig.447

Figure 444: Beginning. Both practitioners stand facing each other in the starting posture for the barehand sequence.

Figure 445: B steps his left leg forward and then his right to punch W in the chest with the right fist.

Figure 446: W counters by sliding the right hand up to deflect the power of the punch. At the same time, W shifts into Shuen Gi Bu.

Figure 447: B slides his left hand under W's arm while shifting the stance to Dsao Pan Bu.

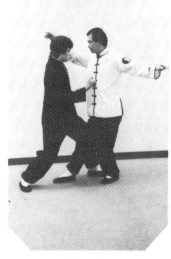

Fig.448

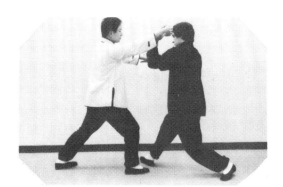

Fig.449

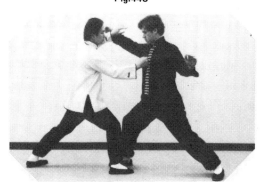

Fig.450

Fig.451

Figure 448: B steps forward with the left leg to punch W.

Figure 449: W counters by sliding his left hand up to deflect the punch while stepping back two paces. B then steps one more pace forward with the right leg.

Figure 450: W slides the right hand away and punches forward.

Figure 451: B shifts his stance to Dsao Pan Bu while deflecting W's punch up with the area between the thumb and forefinger of the left hand.

Figure 452: B steps his left leg behind W and pushes with the shoulder and upper arm.

Figure 453: To counter, W sits back into Ssu Lieu Bu while moving the left hand to B's upper arm.

Figure 454: W slides and pulls B's arm away while raising his right leg and stepping behind B, striking B in the back of the head.

Figure 455: B counters by sitting back and placing his right hand under W's left hand. Next, B spreads his arms open.

Figure 456: B shifts into Deng San Bu to attack W's chest with the left elbow.

Figure 457: W counters by sitting back in Ssu Lieu Bu, sliding his right hand under W's arm to guide B's power to the side.

Figure 458: W shifts to Deng San Bu and attacks B's chest with his upper arm.

Figure 459: B sits back into Ssu Lieu Bu while swinging his right hand under W's attacking arm.

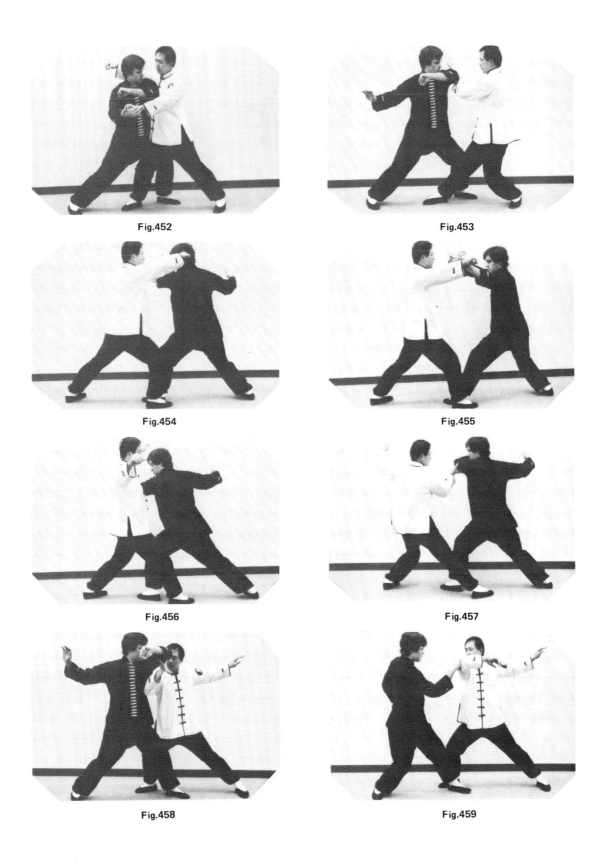

Fig.452

Fig.453

Fig.454

Fig.455

Fig.456

Fig.457

Fig.458

Fig.459

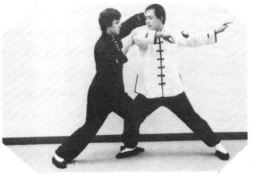

Fig.460

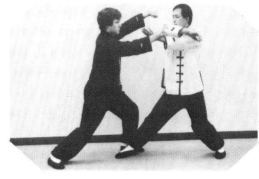

Fig.461

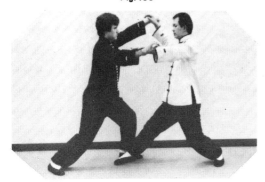

Fig.462

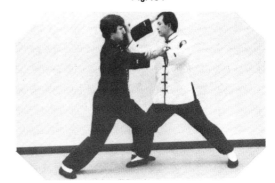

Fig.463

Figure 460: B slides W's arm to the side while stepping the left leg behind W and striking the head with the left fist.

Figure 461: W sits back into Ssu Lieu Bu and slides his left hand up under his right elbow.

Figure 462: W spreads his arms open and slides B's strike away.

Figure 463: W shifts his stance forward into Deng San Bu and strikes down into B's eyebridge with the back of the right fist.

Figure 464: B counters by shifting back into Shuen Gi Bu, left leg forward, and by following W's punching hand down with his left hand.

Figure 465: B steps forward with his right leg to the side of W and cuts at W's neck with the edge of his right palm.

Figure 466: To counter, W pushes B's shoulder.

Figure 467: To avoid being pushed over, B places his left hand on the inside of W's right hand.

Figure 468: B turns his shoulders, making W's hands slip off. B then strikes W's face with the back of the right fist.

Figure 469: W slides his left hand up, sliding B's attack away.

Figure 470: W punches to B's chest with his right fist.

Figure 471: B slides his left hand up to block.

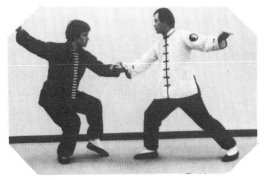

Fig.464

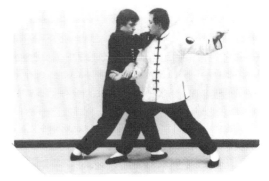

Fig.465

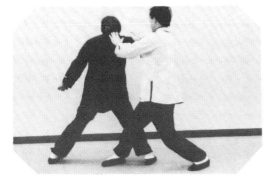

Fig.466

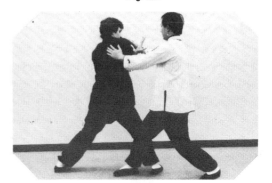

Fig.467

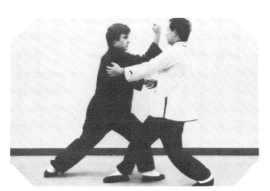

Fig.468

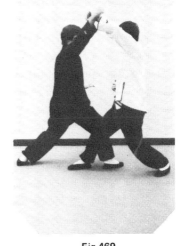

Fig.469

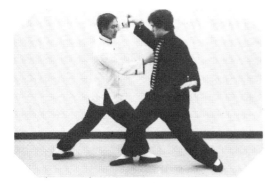

Fig.470

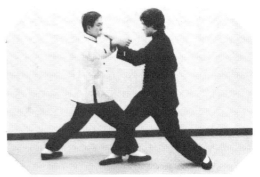

Fig.471

127

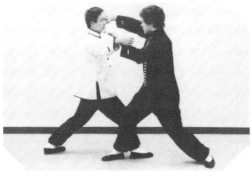

Fig.472

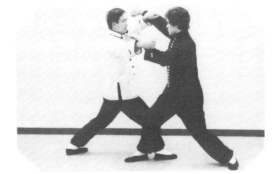

Fig.473

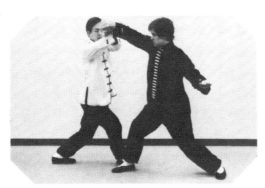

Fig.474

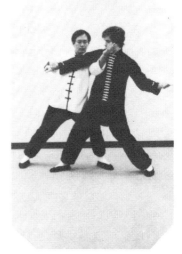

Fig.475

Figure 472: B then swings his right fist down, up, and across to strike W in the temple.

Figure 473: W raises his left arm to block.

Figure 474: W then moves his right hand under and in front of his left hand while turning the legs so the stance is Dsao Pan Bu.

Figure 475: W switches feet and strikes B with the arm under the area of the armpit.

Figure 476: To counter, B uses his left hand to push W's arm away while pulling his own right hand back.

Figure 477: B releases his right hand and punches W's side.

Figure 478: To avoid B's punch, W steps straight back with his left leg while grabbing hold of B's right wrist with his own left hand.

Figure 479: As W steps back, he pulls B while applying pressure on B's elbow with the right arm.

Figure 480: To avoid being brought to the ground, B steps quickly in front of W with both legs together. B places his right hand against his left wrist.

Figure 481: B steps forward with his left leg and pushes W.

Figure 482: To counter B's push, W slides both hands under B's arms while turning the hips to the side away from B's power.

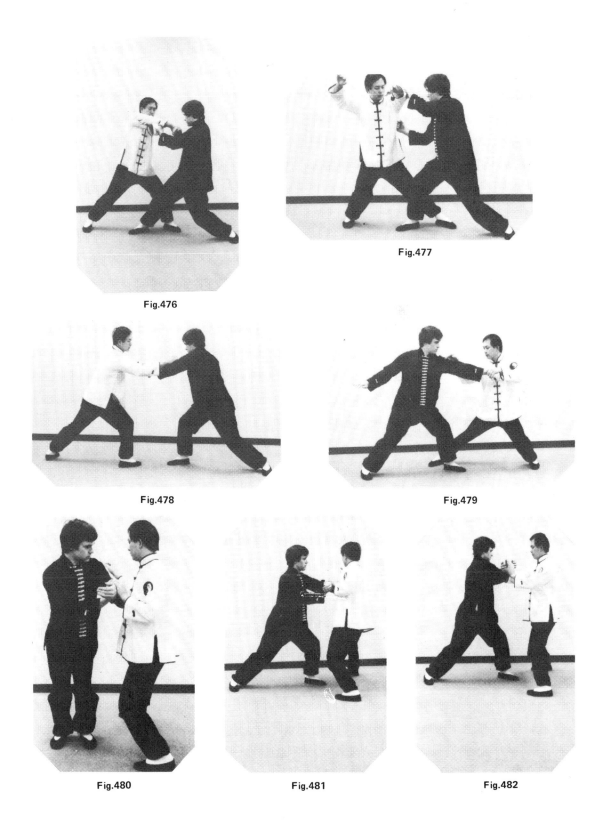

Fig.476

Fig.477

Fig.478

Fig.479

Fig.480

Fig.481

Fig.482

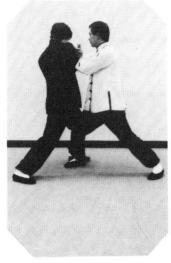

Fig.483

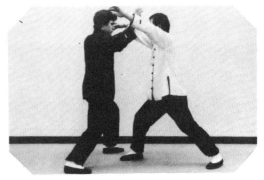

Fig.484

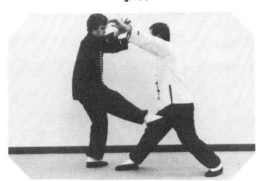

Fig.485

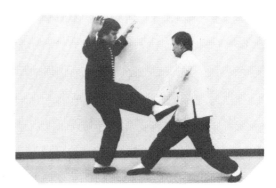

Fig.486

Figure 483: W steps to the right side and pushes B. W's left hand is pressing against his right wrist.

Figure 484: B slides his hands under W's arms and spreads them open to dissolve the push.

Figure 485: Using his right leg, B kicks to W's groin.

Figure 486: Using his left hand, W slides the kick away while also hooking the attacker's leg.

Figure 487: W shifts his stance forward to Deng San Bu and punches B's belly.

Figure 488: B sets his right leg down and slides the punch away with his right hand, circling to the outside to perform the block.

Figure 489: B slaps W's elbow to the side with his left hand.

Figure 490: B steps forward with the right leg and sweeps his right arm into W's head.

Figure 491: W slides B's arm up with his own right. As W guides away B's attacking arm, he attacks B's side with his left palm.

Figure 492: B moves his left hand under W's attacking hand and slides it up.

Figure 493: B then attacks W's side with his right palm.

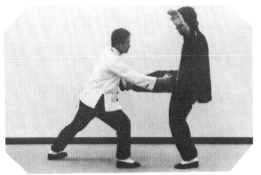

Fig.487

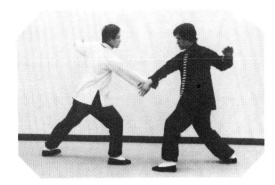

Fig.488

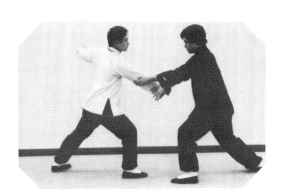

Fig.489

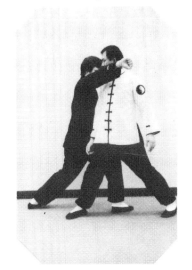

Fig.490

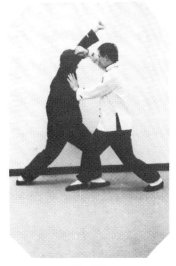

Fig.491

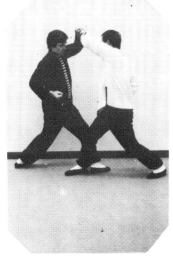

Fig.492

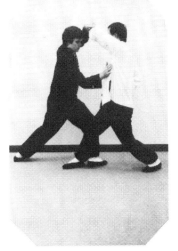

Fig.493

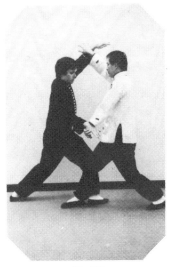

Fig.494

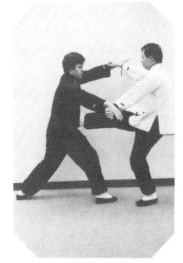

Fig.495

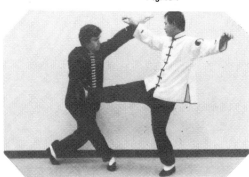

Fig.496

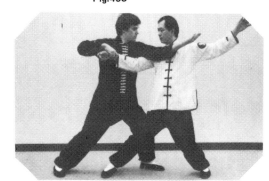

Fig.497

Figure 494: To counter, W moves his right hand up and his left hand down to block the strike.

Figure 495: W hops up and kicks with his right heel.

Figure 496: B turns his legs so the stance is Dsao Pan Bu while sliding the kick away with his right hand.

Figure 497: B steps forward with his left leg, pulls down W's right hand, switches W's hands, and strikes up with his left arm.

Figure 498: W blocks B's arm with his left while pulling his right hand in.

Figure 499: W moves his right leg behind B while pulling on B's left arm. W also applies pressure over B's elbow.

Figure 500: To counter the pull, B steps forward with his right leg while placing his right hand on W's arm.

Figure 501: B next swings his left leg around and applies pressure over W's elbow while also pulling on W's left arm.

Figure 502: W places his right hand under his left forearm, then spreads his arms open.

Figure 503: W steps forward with the right leg and strikes at B's temples with both fists.

Figure 504: To counter, B sits back into Ssu Lieu Bu while sliding his hands down to dissolve W's power away.

Figure 505: B then attempts to push forward with both hands into W's chest. W immediately counters by sliding his hands to the inside to guide B's push away.

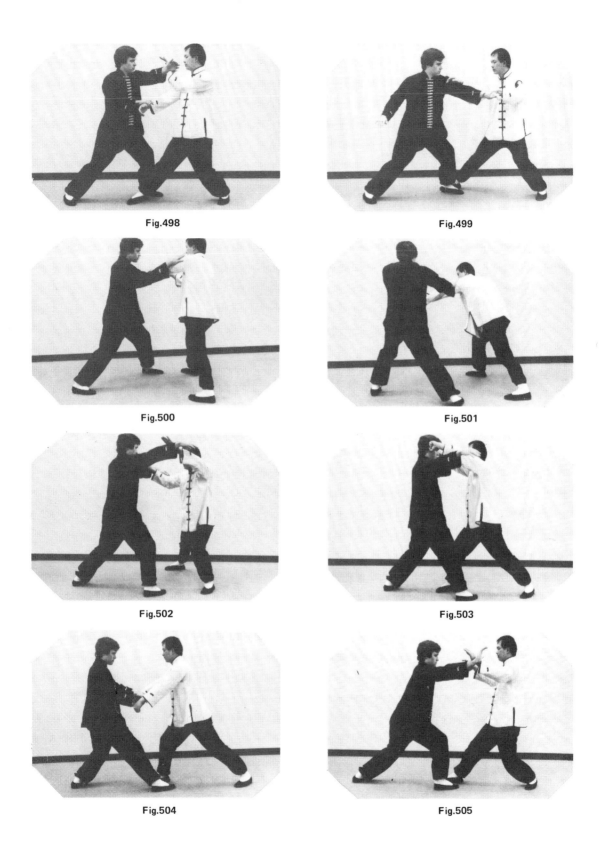

Fig.498

Fig.499

Fig.500

Fig.501

Fig.502

Fig.503

Fig.504

Fig.505

133

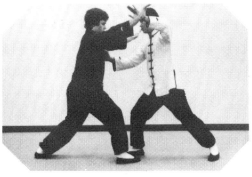

Fig.506

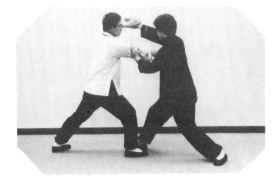

Fig.507

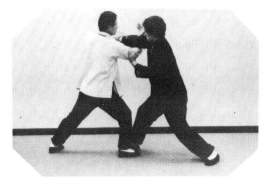

Fig.508

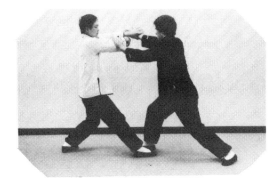

Fig.509

Figure 506: After dissolving B's power, W punches to B's chest with the right fist.

Figure 507: B pushes the punch away with his left palm.

Figure 508: In the act of pushing W's punch away, B has set up W for his next technique. As W's hand is being pushed, W will follow the push in order to hook his right hand under B's elbow. From this position, W can snap B's elbow.

Figure 509: To avoid getting his arm trapped, B pushes W's right arm out.

Figure 510: W spreads his arms open.

Figure 511: W attacks B's chest with the right palm.

Figure 512: To block the strike, B switches the position of his feet while guiding W's left hand down. B uses his left hand to guide W's attack down.

Figure 513: B shifts his stance to Deng San Bu and strikes W's chest with his left palm.

Figure 514: W raises his arms and guides the attack away while sitting back in Ssu Lieu Bu.

Figure 515: W shifts his stance forward into Deng San Bu and strikes B's chest with his right elbow.

Figure 516: B sits back and slides his left hand under W's elbow to guide the attack to the side.

Figure 517: B switches feet and swings his right arm into W's head.

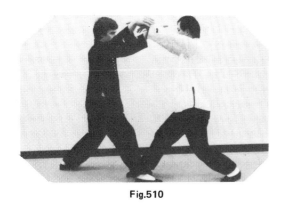

Fig.510

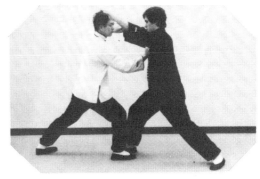

Fig.511

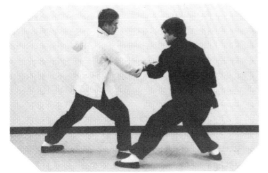

Fig.512

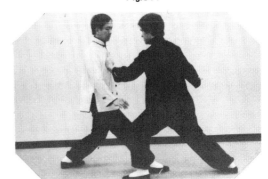

Fig.513

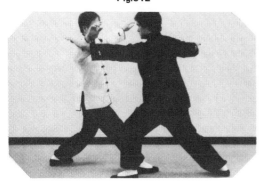

Fig.514

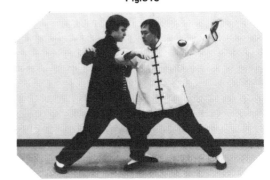

Fig.515

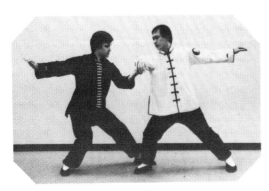

Fig.516

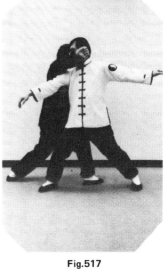

Fig.517

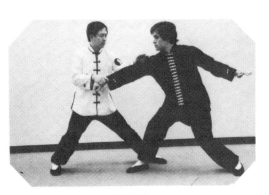

Fig.518

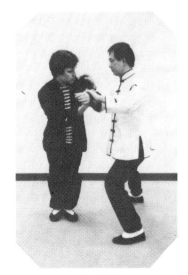

Fig.519

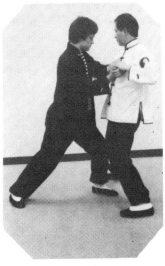

Fig.520

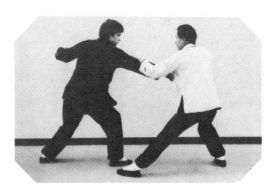

Fig.521

Figure 518: W slides his right hand up and grabs B's hand while also neutralizing the attack. W then moves his right leg back and pulls B.

Figure 519: B quickly brings both feet together in front of W.

Figure 520: B steps in with his left leg and pushes W.

Figure 521: W slides his hands uner B's arms and steps back with his right leg while pulling B.

Figure 522: To counter W's pull, B places his left hand under W's left hand.

Figure 523: Next, B slides his right hand away and strikes at W's head while stepping to the side with the right leg.

Figure 524: W grabs B's left wrist with his left hand and steps back with the left leg while pulling B. W's right arm exerts pressure on B's elbow.

Figure 525: B steps in front of W with both legs.

Figure 526: B pushes W. B's right hand is on his left wrist.

Figure 527: To dissolve B's push, W slides his left hand under B's arms to guide the power away.

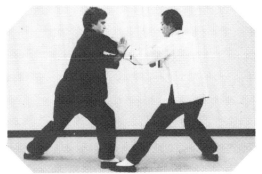

Fig.522

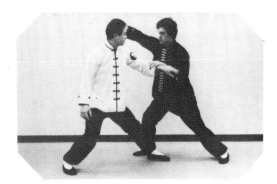

Fig.523

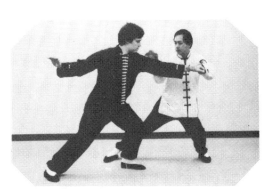

Fig.524

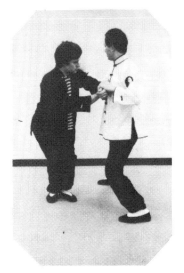

Fig.525

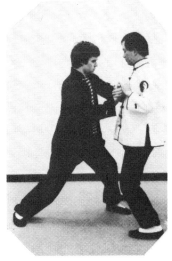

Fig.526

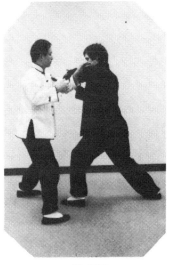

Fig.527

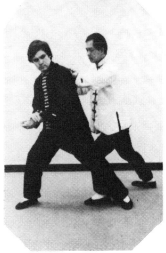

Fig.528

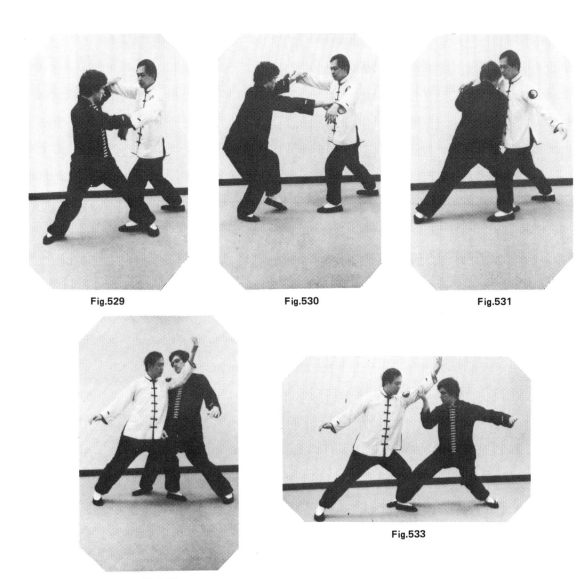

Fig.529 Fig.530 Fig.531

Fig.532

Fig.533

Figure 528: W swings his left leg around and pushes B's back.

Figure 529: To counter, B spreads W's arms apart by swinging his right hand up and then down, and his left hand straight up.

Figure 530: B turns his body to face W while shifting his stance to Shuen Gi Bu, left foot on its toes.

Figure 531: B steps forward with the right leg and rams W's chest with his shoulder.

Figure 532: To avoid the shoulder strike, W switches feet and swings his left arm into B's chest. W's feet are in front of B.

Figure 533: B sits back and guides the attack away by swinging the right hand up.

Figure 534: B shifts his stance to Deng San Bu and uses his right elbow to attack W's chest.

Figure 535: W slides his left hand down and dissovles the attack to the side.

Figure 536: W hops up and kicks B with his left knee.

Figure 537: To counter the knee kick, B quickly sits back and pulls down on both of W's arms. By pulling down on the arms, W cannot kick.

Figure 538: W raises his hands up and kicks with the left heel. To send off the kick, W hops.

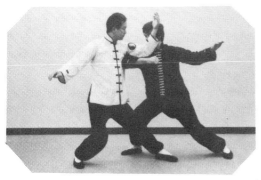

Fig.534

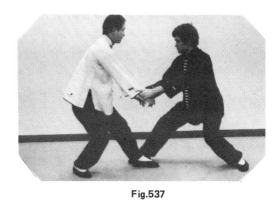

Fig.535

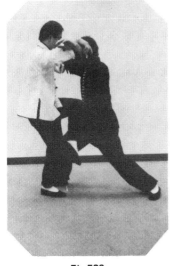

Fig.536

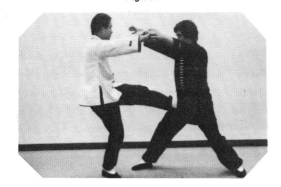

Fig.537

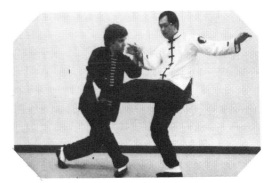

Fig.538

Fig.539

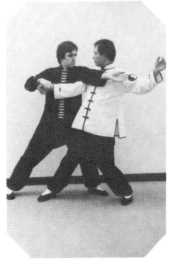

Fig.540

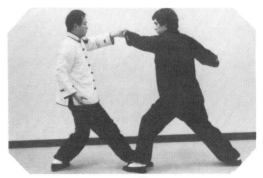

Fig.541

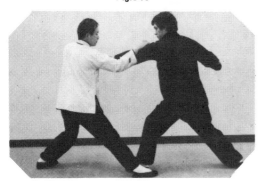

Fig.542

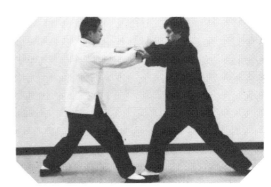

Fig.543

Figure 539: To avoid W's attack, B turns his legs so his stance is Dsao Pan Bu while hooking the kicking leg. At the same time, B hooks W's right hand down.

Figure 540: B steps forward with the left leg and strikes up at W with his left arm. B's right hand grabs W's right hand as B's left arm swings to strike. B stands behind W.

Figure 541: W sits back in Ssu Lieu Bu while pulling his right arm in and pushing B's left arm away.

Figure 542: W steps behind B and pulls while exerting pressure on B's elbow.

Figure 543: To counter W's pull, B slides his right hand under W's wrist to push w's grip away.

Figure 544: B raises W's hand and kicks with his right leg.

Figure 545: W swings his left hand up and his right hand down to block the kick.

Figure 546: B retreats his right leg and slides the left hand up, thus freeing the right hand.

Figure 547: B sets his right leg down and kicks with the left leg.

Figure 548: W swings the right hand and the left hand down to block the kick.

Figure 549: B retreats his left leg and crosses his right hand over his left.

Figure 550: B uses his right hand to push W's right hand to the side.

140

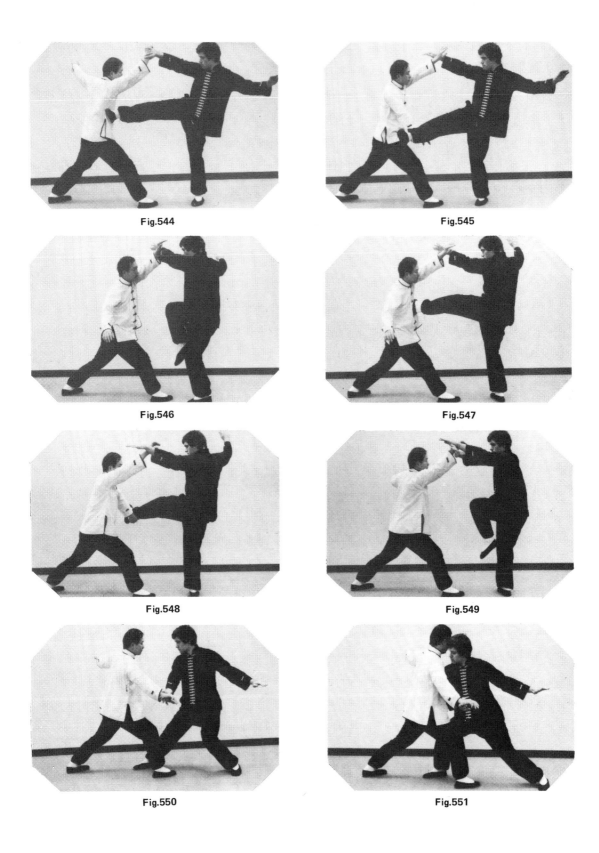

Fig.544

Fig.545

Fig.546

Fig.547

Fig.548

Fig.549

Fig.550

Fig.551

141

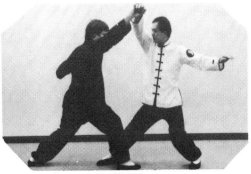

Fig.552

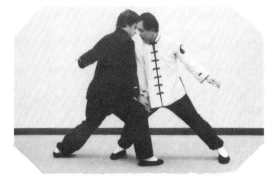

Fig.553

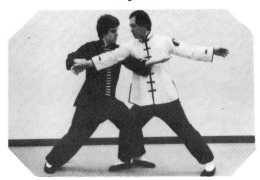

Fig.554

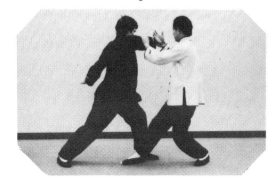

Fig.555

Figure 551: B moves into W to ram his chest with his shoulder.

Figure 552: W sits back and grabs B's right hand while swinging his arm in a big clockwise circle.

Figure 553: Once the motion of the circle has come close to completion, W can use his shoulder to hit B's shoulder blade in the back. To counter this move, B turns his shoulders so that it rams into W's shoulder.

Figure 554: B moves his right leg back and attacks W's chest by swinging his left forearm under W's arm.

Figure 555: W pulls his right arm back while shifting to Ssu Lie Bu.

Figure 556: To begin the counter, B slides his left hand under W's left hand.

Figure 557: B moves his right leg forward and attacks W's chest, using his right forearm.

Figure 558: W uses his left hand to grab and pull B's left hand. W's right hand assists in the pull.

Figure 559: B puts his right hand under his left wrist and spreads his arms open.

Figure 560: B attacks by pressing forward into W's chest.

142

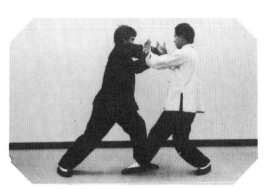

Fig.556

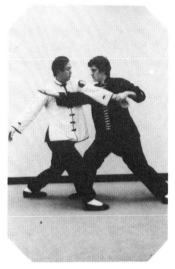

Fig.557.

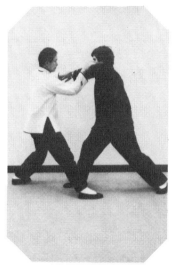

Fig.558

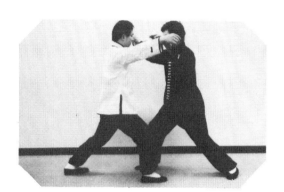

Fig.559

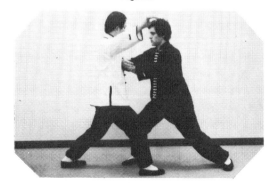

Fig.560

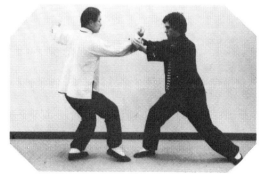

Fig.561

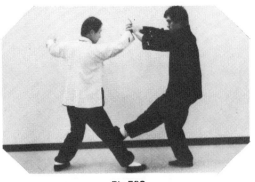

Fig.562

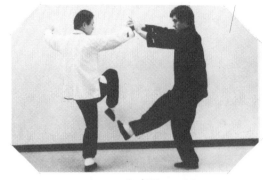

Fig.563

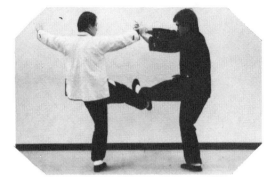

Fig.564

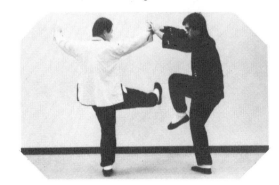

Fig.565

Figure 561: To counter, W swings his right hand down and up to slide the attack away while shifting the stance into Shuen Gi Bu.

Figure 562: B grabs W's hand and then kicks at W's knee with the left heel.

Figure 563: W raises his right leg to avoid the kick.

Figure 564: W uses his right leg to hook B's kicking leg up in order to trip him.

Figure 565: To avoid the hook, B withdraws his right leg.

Figure 566: B sets his left leg down, then swings his right leg into W's back.

Figure 567: W counters by quickly switching feet, pulling down B's right arm, then attacking B's chest by a forearm strike from underneath the arm.

Figure 568: B turns his body clockwise while shuffling his legs until his left leg is in front of W. B then strikes W's chest with the left palm.

Figure 569: W moves the right leg forward while the left leg swings back. As W is moving, he swings his left hand down and up in order to slide B's attack away. After sliding the attack away, W grabs B's arm and attacks the chest with a forearm strike from underneath the arm.

Figure 570: B pulls his left arm back while pushing W's right arm away.

Figure 571: B moves his left leg behind W and strikes W's head with his left fist.

Figure 572: W places his left hand under B's right wrist and spreads his arms open to block the punch. As W spreads his hands open, he shifts stance into Shuen Gi Bu.

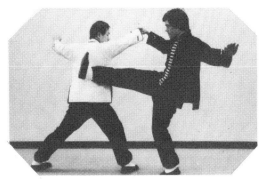

Fig.566

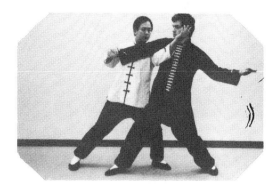

Fig.567

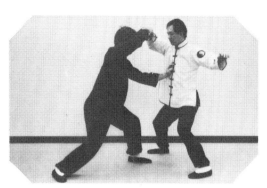

Fig.568

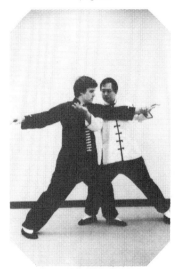

Fig.569

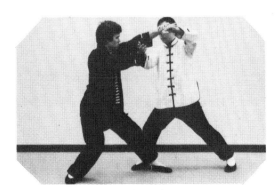

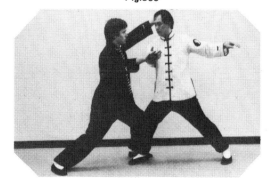

Fig.570

Fig.571

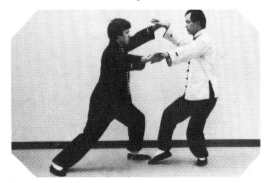

Fig.572

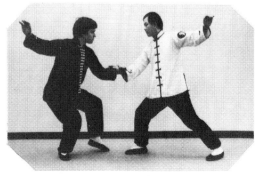

Fig.573

145

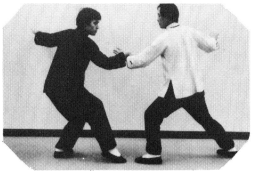 

Fig.574

Fig.575

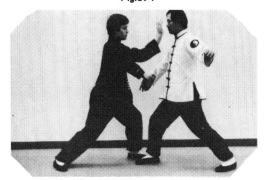

Fig.576

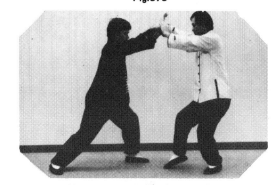

Fig.577

Figure 573: W strikes to B's eyebridge with the back of his right fist as W shifts his stance to Deng San Bu. To counter, B sits back in Shuen Gi Bu and guides W's arm down with his left hand.

Figure 574: W then steps forward with his left leg to strike B in the face with the left palm. B counters by moving his left leg back so the stance is Shuen Gi Bu again. At the same time that B moves back, he uses his right hand to guide W's attack down.

Figure 575: W steps forward with his right leg and strikes at B's face with his right palm. To counter, B moves his right leg back so the stance is Shuen Gi Bu while using his left hand to guide the attack down.

Figure 576: B shifts his stance into Deng San Bu while striking at W's face with his right palm.

Figure 577: W slides his hands up to dissolve the attack, while shifting the stance to Shuen Gi Bu.

Figure 578: W kicks B's groin with his right leg.

Figure 579: B grabs W's right hand and pulls W, thus preventing him from kicking. B has his left palm over the right wrist.

Figure 580: W pulls back up to counter B's move. W's left hand aids in the pull.

Figure 581: B pulls down once again.

Figure 582: W pulls up again, then uses his left palm to strike under B's right arm in the chest area.

Figure 583: B then pulls W's right arm, exerting pressure over the elbow.

Figure 584: W grabs B's right hand with his right hand and pulls. W's left hand helps with the pull.

146

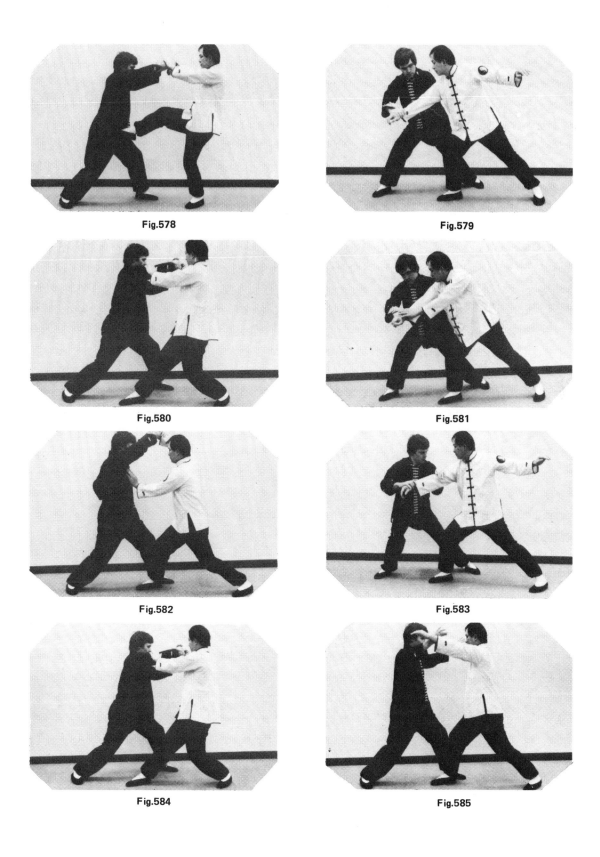

Fig.578

Fig.579

Fig.580

Fig.581

Fig.582

Fig.583

Fig.584

Fig.585

147

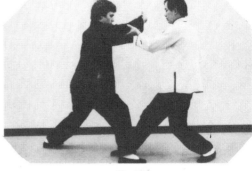

Fig.586

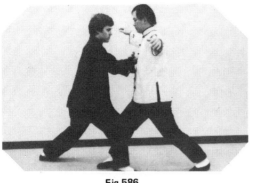

Fig.587

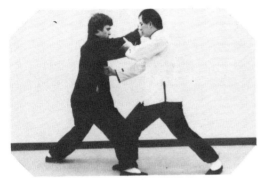

Fig.588

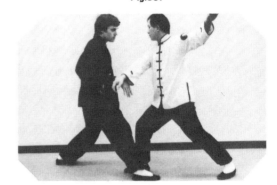

Fig.589

Figure 585: B places his left hand under his right wrist. B then spreads his arms open to neutralize the pull.

Figure 586 B switches feet and strikes W in the chest with his left hand pressing on the inside of his right wrist.

Figure 587: W slides his left hand under B's arm to slide the attack away.

Figure 588: W punches to B's midsection with the right fist.

Figure 589: B slides his right hand down to guide the punch away.

Figure 590: B uses the fingers of his left hand to attack W's eyes.

Figure 591: W moves his right hand up and his left hand down. The right hand blocks the attack.

Figure 592: W pushes into B's chest with both hands.

Figure 593: B shifts his stance to Shuen Gi Bu and slides W's push away by sliding his hands to an inside position.

Figure 594: Both sides move their right legs back while raising their arms, palms down to chest level.

Figure 595: Both sides lower their arms, thus assuming the original position.

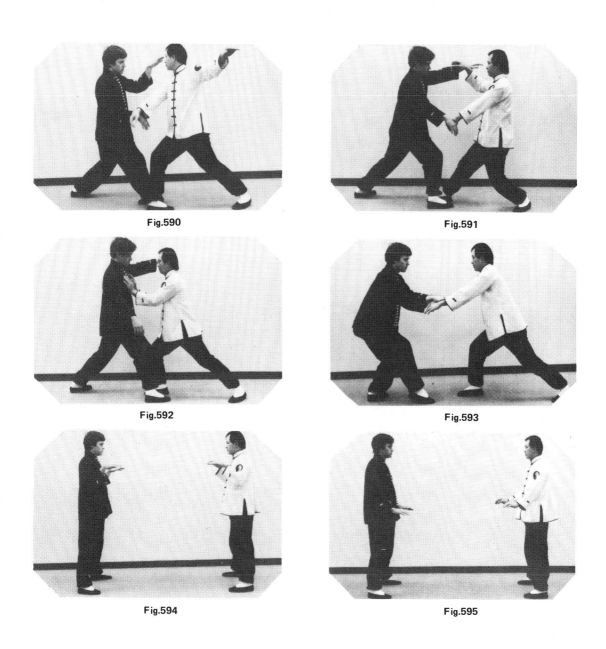

Fig.590

Fig.591

Fig.592

Fig.593

Fig.594

Fig.595

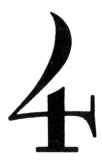

TAI CHI NARROW BLADE SWORD

One of the highest achievements in Tai Chi is the use of the narrow blade sword. As was mentioned in Chapter 1, the narrow blade sword, the king of the short weapons, requires at least ten years of Tai Chi training before it can be started. Although the Tai Chi narrow blade sword is usually begun in the tenth year of practice, this book will present the Tai Chi sword for the purpose of information. In addition, the individual who is interested in Tai Chi for its health aspect can perform the sword sequence as another method of exercise.

There are basically two reasons why a Tai Chi martial artist must practice ten years before starting instruction in the narrow blade sword. First, because of the construction and techniques of the narrow blade sword, blocking requires the use of soft, non violent, power. The defensive techniques of the sword are very much like those of the barehand maneuvers; both require the ability to stick to an opponent while avoiding the enemy's attack. Thus, the Tai Chi martial artist must be proficient in the methods of neutralizing an opponent's power before he starts sword training.

The second reason the Tai Chi martial artist must train for ten years before staring the narrow blade sword is that the techniques of the weapon require the smooth circulation of Chi to all parts of the body. Because the Tai Chi narrow blade sword is very flexible, the martial artist must have the ability to pass his Chi into the sword to momentarily harden it. To pass Chi into the sword requires Grand Circulation. To help the Chi into the sword, Tai Chi practitioners use a special form called the Secret Sword Hand on the arm that is not holding the sword (Figure 1). The Secret Sword Hand symmetrically balances Chi circulation so the Chi can enter the sword. This hand form is also used for cavity press during combat.

In actual construction, the narrow blade sword is flexible and sharp in different areas. The top third of the blade (Figure 2A) is extremely thin and razor sharp. The top third is never used for blocking because it can be dented very easily. Instead, this sharp part is used only for attack. The middle third of the blade (Figure 2B) is thicker and less sharp than the top third. This part of the blade is used for sliding, guiding away, sticking, and cutting. The bottom third (Figure 2C) is very thick and unsharpened. The bottom third is usually used for situations when violent power is needed. Thus, because of the unique construction of the sword, the Tai Chi martial artist will attempt to keep his opponent in the middle and long range for proper usage.

Once again, due to the construction of the narrow blade sword and the techniques emphasized by Tai Chi stylists, there are only a few effective methods of using the sword. Basically, the Tai Chi student can slide, sting or stab, deflect cut (sliding and cutting in the same motion), slash, or chop while handling the sword. Most of the motions are done with fluidity and extreme speed. But to properly use each movement of the sword, the stylist must be capable of smooth locomotion. Without the correct use of the legs, each motion of the sword can be wasted. In fact, the ultimate goal of the Tai Chi swordsman is to successfully attack by never touching the weapon of the opponent through the use of deceptively quick steps.

After the Tai Chi martial artist learns the narrow blade sword sequence, he will go on to exercises that serve the same function as pushing hands, but which are done with a sword. These drills are called fighting forms. The Tai Chi student must practice and become proficient in the fighting forms because they will train all the important abilities needed for free fighting: smooth Chi flow into the sword, fluid and alive movement, an understanding of the opponent's power, an ability to adhere, expertise in sword

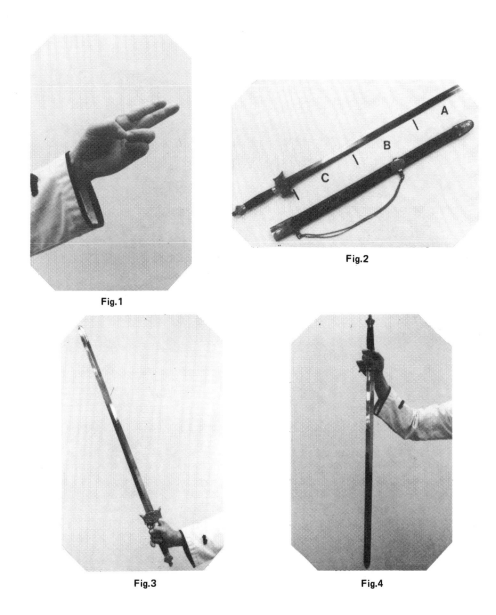

Fig.1

Fig.2

Fig.3

Fig.4

technique, and proper defense. In this book, 11 sword fighting forms will be shown and explained: six for right side attack and defense, and five for left side attack and defense. Later, experienced Tai Chi stylists can develop their own fighting forms. Once all the requirements are met, the student proceeds to unrestricted fighting.

In performing the slow motion Tai Chi sword sequence, a few precautionary points must be noted. When holding the sword, the hand must remain loose. Although the sword is held loosely, it is always under strict control. The two methods of holding the sword are shown in Figures 3 and 4. Second, concentrate on passing the Chi into the sword—this aspect will take time and energy to achieve. Third, co-ordinate all the forms with deep breathing. The order of the breaths will be in the description of the sequence. Like the barehand sequence, the sword forms must be done slowly in order to get the full benefits of this elegant and ancient weapon sequence. Finally, observe all the points that were mentioned for correct practice of the Tai Chi barehand sequence such as placing the tongue on the roof of the mouth, relaxation, keeping the elbows low, keeping the spine straight, etc. With patience and practice, the practitioner can make the Tai Chi sword sequence a useful and beautiful series of techniques for health or defense.

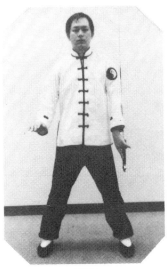
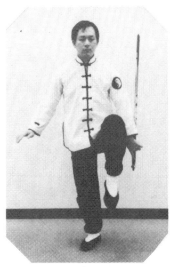
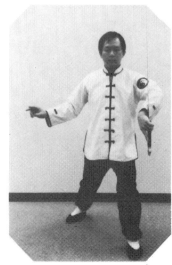

| Fig.5 | Fig.6 | Fig.7 |

Yang's Narrow Blade Sword Sequence (Appendix B)

1. Beginning (Ch'i Shih)
Figure 5: (N) The sword is held at the left side and the right palm faces down. Inhale and exhale.

2. Step Forward and Close with Sword (Shang Pu Ho Chien Shih)
Figure 6: (N) Raise your left knee. Begin to inhale.

Figure 7: (N) Step forward and slightly off to the side with your left leg. The right hand forms the Secret Sword Hand. Complete inhalation.

Figure 8: (N) Bring your right leg forward while lifting its knee. Set your right leg down so the stance is Ma Bu. Swing your right hand Secret Sword to your left wrist while bringing your left arm, with the sword, to the front of your body. Exhale.

3. Fairy Shows the Way (Hsien Jen Chih Lu)
Figure 9: (W) Turn your body to W while changing stanced to Shuen Gi Bu. Swing the sword across your body, and raise your right hand. Inhale.

Figure 9A: As an opponent attempts to stab the abdomen, the defender slides away the attacker's weapon.

Figure 10: (W) Shift the stance to Deng San Bu and move the right hand forward at chest level. Exhale.

Figure 10A: After sliding the opponent's sword away, the defender attacks with the Secret Sword Hand.

4. Three Rings Envelope the Moon (San Fuan T'ao Yeuh)
Figure 11: (W) Make a small clockwise circle with your right hand. Begin to inhale. This technique is used to block a punch.

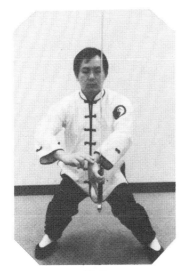

Fig.8

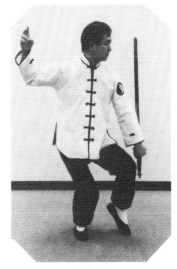

Fig.9

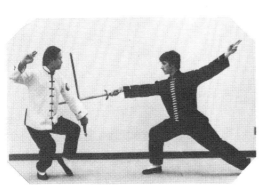

Fig.9A

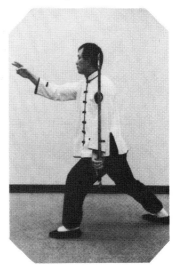

Fig.10

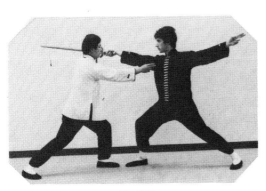

Fig.10A

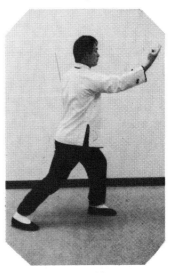

Fig.11

153

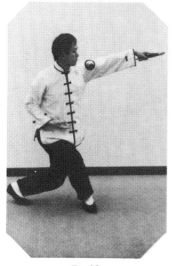

Fig.12

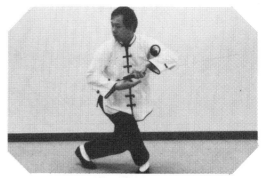

Fig.13

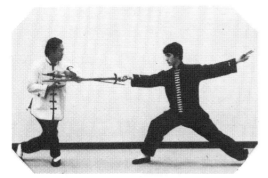

Fig.13A

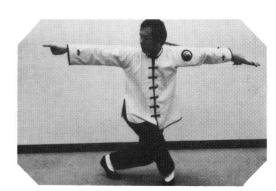

Fig.14

Figure 12: (W) Step forward your your right leg into Dsao Pan Bu. Swing the sword to the front with the handle pointed out. Retreat your right hand to your waist. Complete inhalation.

Figure 13: (W) Bring the sword to the front of your body; at the same time move your right hand to the underside of the sword. Begin to exhale. Face looks E.

Figure 13A: As the opponent stabs, the defender slides the weapon away.

Figure 14: (W) Swing both arms down and up. The upper body faces N and the face looks E. Complete exhalation.

Figure 14A: After blocking in 13A, the defender slides the attacker's sword down and away in order to attack with the handle of the sword.

Figure 15: (W) Step with your left leg forward into Deng San Bu while swinging your right hand over your left. Inhale.

Figure 16: (E) Switch the sword to your right hand and turn 180 degrees clockwise while sliding the sword to knee level. The left hand stays in touch with your right wrist. Exhale.

Figure 16A: The defender dodges the attack and cuts the enemy's knee.

5. Big Chief Star (Da Kuai Hsing)

Figure 17: (E) Raise the sword while beginning to draw your left leg up. Inhale.

Figure 18: (W) Raise your left knee while turning 180 degrees counterclockwise. The sword arches above the head during the turn. While your body is turning, your left hand pushes forward from your chest. Exhale.

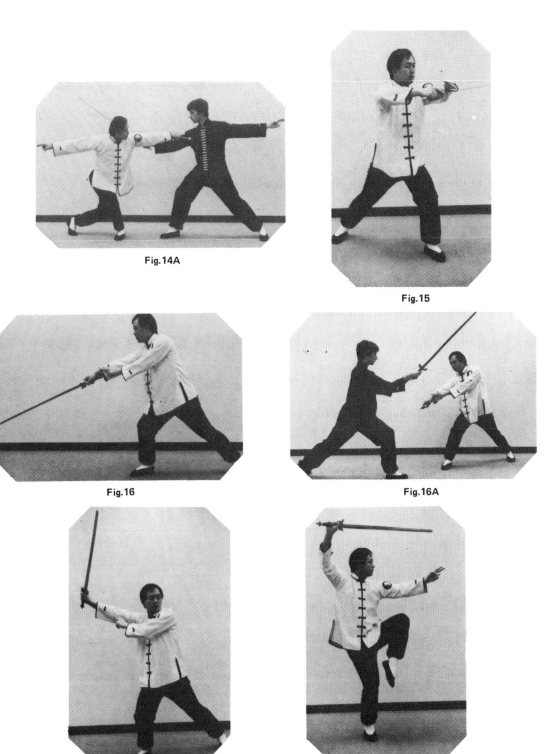

Fig.14A

Fig.15

Fig.16

Fig.16A

Fig.17

Fig.18

155

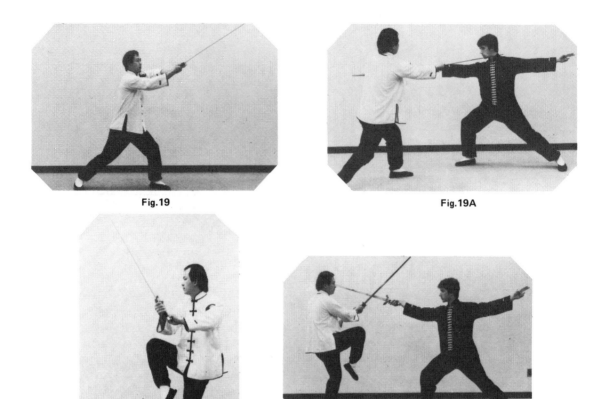

Fig.19

Fig.19A

Fig.20

Fig.20A

6. Swallow Seizes Water (Yen Tzu Ch'ao Shui)
> Figure 19: (SW) Step your left leg down into Deng San Bu and slide the sword up slightly. Your left hand touches your right wrist. Inhale and exhale.
> Figure 19A: As the opponent stabs forward, the defender moves to the side and slides his sword across the neck of the attacker. This is not a hacking motion, but a foward slide.

7. Left Sweep: Right Sweep (Tso Yu Lan Sao)
> Figure 20: (SW) Raise your right knee while raising the sword so that the flat part faces the practitioner. Inhale.
> Figure 20A: The defender slides away an attack to the upper body with the lower third of the sword.
> Figure 21: (NW) Step your right leg down to the NW while sliding the sword forward. The stance is Deng San Bu and the sword is perpendicular to the body. Exhale.
> Figure 21A: After blocking in 20A, the defender moves in to cut the attacker.
> Figure 22: (NW) Raise your left knee up while moving the sword up so the palm of the sword hand faces to the side. Inhale.
> Figure 22A: The defender slides away an attack from the outside position.
> Figure 23: (SW) Step your left leg down to SW and slide the sword forward. The stance is Deng San Bu and the sword is perpendicular to the body. Exhale.
> Figure 23A: After sliding away the opponent's sword, the defender steps in to attack.

156

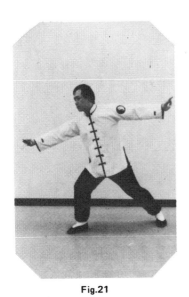

Fig.21

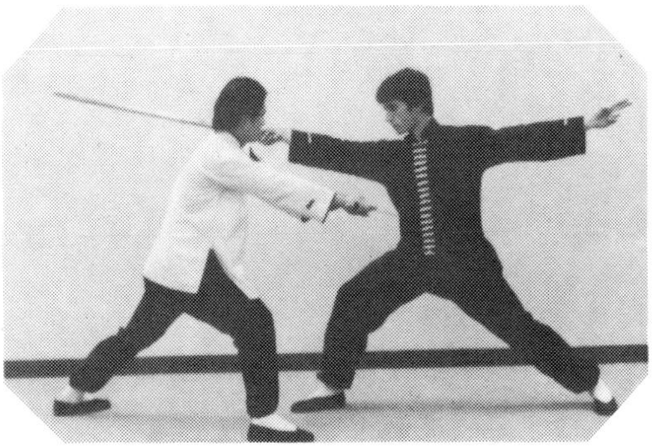

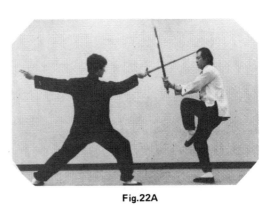

Fig.21A

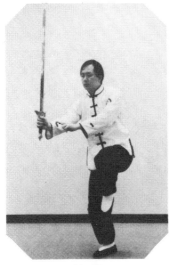

Fig.22

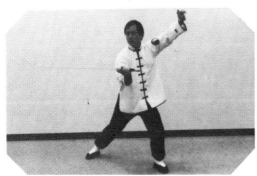

Fig.22A

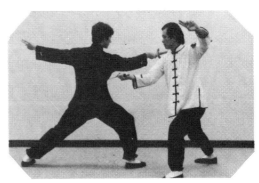

Fig.23

Fig.23A

157

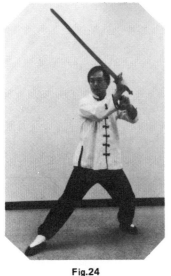

Fig.24

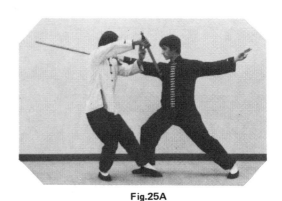

Fig.24A

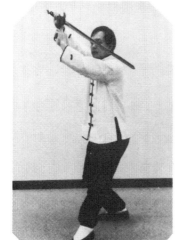

Fig.25

Fig.25A

8. Little Chief Star (Hsiao Kuai Hsing)

Figure 24: (NW) Raise your right leg up and set it down to face NW. At the same time, raise the sword up so the palm of your hand holding it faces in. Inhale.

Figure 24A: The defender slides the attack up with the lower third of the sword.

Figure 25: (NW) Step forward with your left leg into Shuen Gi Bu while swinging the sword back, down, forward, and up. The hand gripping the sword is above the blade. Exhale.

Figure 25A: After blocking, the defender steps forward and slices up into the opponent.

9. Yellow Bee Enters the Hole (Huang Fong Zoo Don)

Figure 26: (NW) Step back with your left leg. Inhale.

Figure 27: (SE) Turn your body 180 degrees counterclockwise into Deng San Bu while pushing the sword forward and down. Exhale.

Figure 27A: As the opponent begins a high attack, the defender stabs low.

10. Spirit Cat Catches the Mouse (Ling Mao Pu Su)

Figure 28: (SE) Sweep your right leg forward and up while turning the sword up. As the sword is being turned up, bring it close to the body. Inhale.

Figure 28A: As the attacker stabs, the defender slides the sword away.

Figure 29: (SE) Step down with your right leg and jump off it; alternately raise both knees while in the air. While in the air, move the sword forward, up, and back in a circular motion. Exhale.

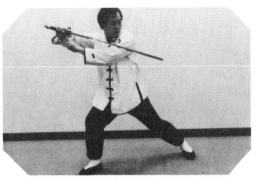

Fig.26

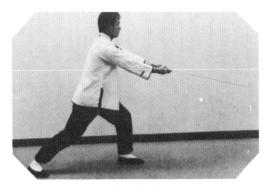

Fig.27

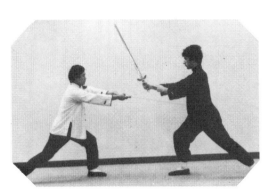

Fig.27A

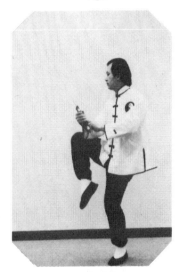

Fig.28

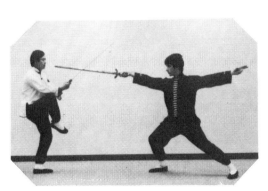

Fig.28A

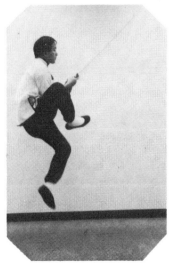

Fig.29

159

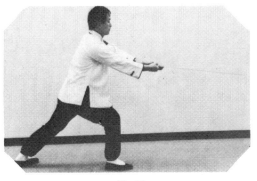

Fig.30

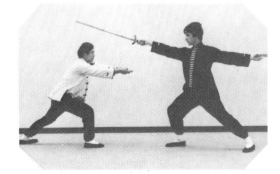

Fig.30A

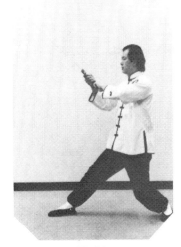

Fig.31

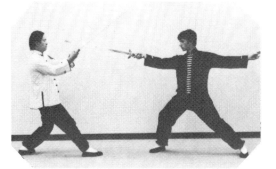

Fig31A

Figure 30: (SE) Land in Deng San Bu, right leg forward. As the landing is made, push the sword down. Complete exhalation.

Figure 30A: After blocking, the defender chases his opponent and stabs him low.

11. **Dragonfly Touches Water (Ching T'ing Tien Shui)**

Figure 31: (SE) Sit back into Ssu Lieu Bu and raise the sword up in a circular motion. Inhale.

Figure 31A: The defender slides away an attack to his upper body with the lower edge of the sword.

Figure 32: (SE) Bring your arm in and push the sword down and forward while shifting the stance to Deng San Bu. Exhale. The motion of the sword is the same as in Figure 29.

12. **Swallow Enters the Nest (Yen Tzu Noo Ch'ao)**

Figure 33: (N) Slide your right leg back 45 degrees counterclockwise so the front of your body is facing directly N. The stance is Shuen Gi Bu. At the same time that your leg is sliding, turn the sword hand clockwise so your palm faces in and the sword points E. Bring the sword hand up to the face. Inhale.

Figure 33A: As the opponent attacks, the defender steps back into Shuen Gi Bu and slides the attacker's sword to the side. The block is made near the lower edge of the sword.

Figure 34: (E) Shift the stance into Deng San Bu while sliding the sword up, back, and straight forward so the sword handle is in front of the blade. Face looks S.

Figure 34A: After the defender slides the attack away, he steps forward and cuts under the attacker's arm.

Figure 35: (E) Spin 360 degrees counterclockwise on your left leg while keeping the sword stationary. Your right leg is lifted. Begin to inhale.

160

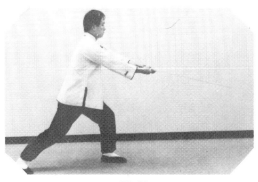

Fig.32

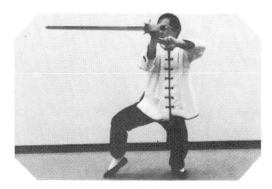

Fig.33

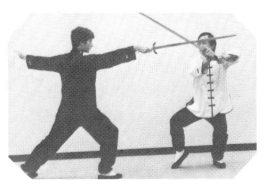

Fig.33A

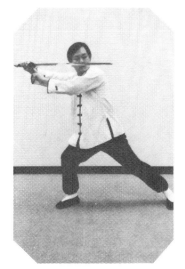

Fig.34

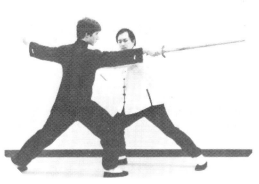

Fig.34A

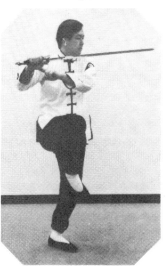

Fig.35

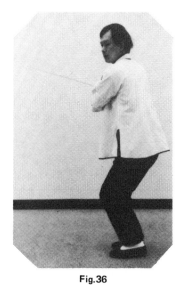

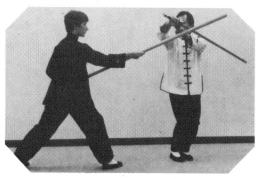

Fig.36A

Fig.36

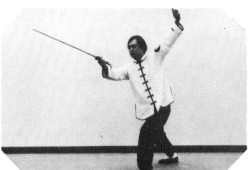

Fig.37

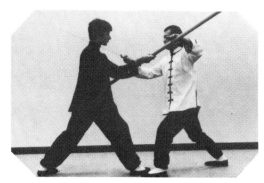

Fig.37A

Figure 36: (E) Set the right leg down and complete inhalation.

figure 36A: This technique is used against attacks which use a long rod. As the opponent stings with his rod, the defender slides the attack away by whirling around. The lower edge of the sword guides the rod away as the turn is made.

Figure 37: (NE) Step with the left leg off to the side, NE, and slide the sword up. The stance is Deng San Bu. Exhale.

Figure 37A: After turning in Figure 36A, the defender steps in and cuts the opponent's neck.

13. Phoenix Spreads Its Wings (Fong Huang Shuang Chan Ch'ih)

Figure 38: (SE) Turn 90 degrees clockwise into Ma Bu while bringing your left hand to the sword. Inhale.

Figure 39: (SW) Turn another 90 degrees clockwise into Deng San Bu while swinging the sword up, palms pointing up. Your left hand retreats to the rear. Exhale.

Figure 39A: The defender dodges an attack and swings the sword up into the opponent's back.

14. Right Whirlwind (Yu Shuen Fong)

Figure 40: (SW) Bring your left leg up and shift the stance to Shuen Gi Bu. While shifting stance, make a small clockwise circle with the handle of the sword, at the same time that the end of the sword remains fixed at one point. To understand the motion of the sword, the practitioner can press his weapon against a wall and only move the handle in a circle. The wrists must be flexible to make the motion properly. Inhale and exhale.

Figure 40A: As the opponent stabs, the defender jumps to the side and circles his sword over the attacker's wrist. As the blade circles, the defender cuts into the opponent's wrist.

Figure 41: (SW) Bring your legs together and begin the previous sword motion again. Inhale.

Figure 42: (SW) Shift the stance to Shuen Gi Bu and complete the previously described sword motion. Exhale.

Figure 43: (SW) Repeat Figure 40. Begin to inhale.

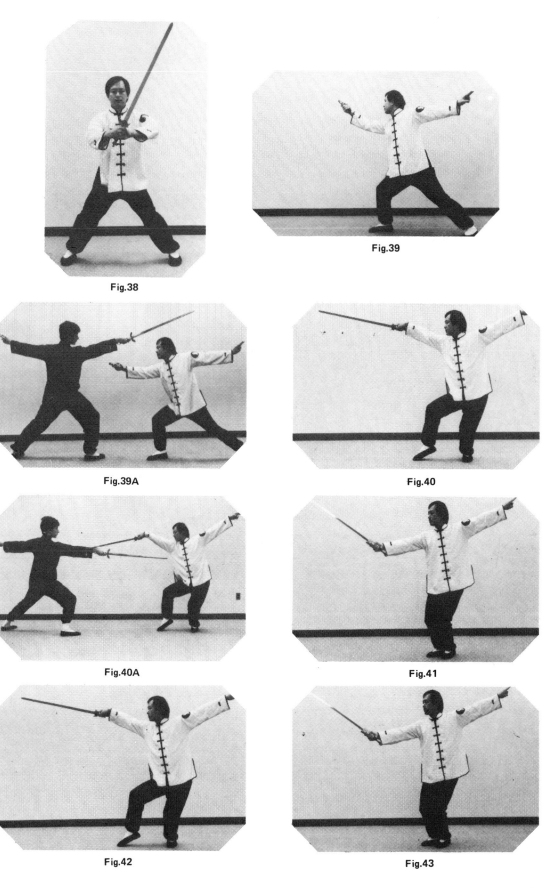

Fig.38

Fig.39

Fig.39A

Fig.40

Fig.40A

Fig.41

Fig.42

Fig.43

163

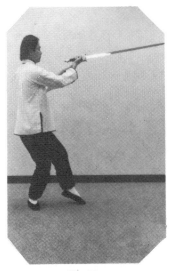

Fig.44

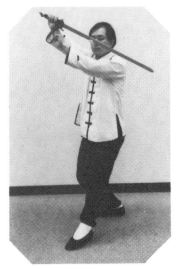

Fig.45

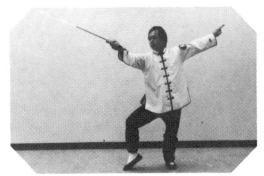

Fig.46

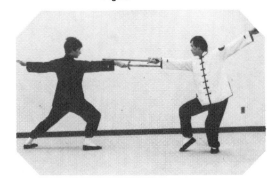

Fig.46A

15. Little Chief Star (Hsiao Kuai Hsing)

Figure 44: (SW) From the previous form, circle the sword up in a continuous motion while shifting the stance to Shuen Gi Bu, left leg forward. Complete inhalation.

Figure 45: (SW) Circle the sword up, back, down, forward and up. Exhale.

16. Left Whirlwind (Tso Shuen Fong)

Figure 46: (SW) Step your left leg back, shifting the stance to Shuen Gi Bu, and circle the handle of the sword in a counterclockwise motion, while keeping the tip of the sword fixed at a point. This is the same type of motion as in Right Whirlwind, except that the sword moves counterclockwise. Begin inhalation.

Figure 46A: As the opponent stabs, the defender moves to the outside and cuts down on the attacker's wrist. Same as Figure 40A, except the defender moves to a different side.

Figure 47: (SW) Set the right foot down and move backwards with your left leg. As your legs are moving, the sword begins the motion described in Figure 46. Complete inhalation.

Figure 48: (SW) Draw your front leg in so the stance is Shuen Gi Bu. Complete the sword motion. Exhale.

Figure 49: (SW) Set your right foot down and move your left leg back while beginning the previous sword motion. Begin to inhale.

17. Wait For the Fish (Teng Yu Shih)

Figure 50: (W) Draw your right leg up into Shuen Gi Bu while raising the sword up from the previous form. Your left hand touches the right wrist. The sword is pointing W. Complete inhalation.

Figure 50A: The defender slides the opponent's sword away.

Figure 51: (W) Keep the sword pointed W and slide it down. The left hand is extended back. Exhale.

Figure 51A: After blocking, the defender stabs the opponent in the belly.

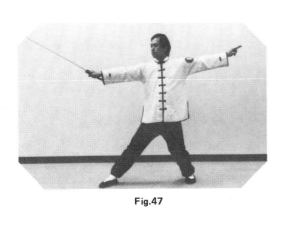

Fig.47

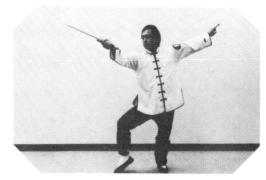

Fig.48

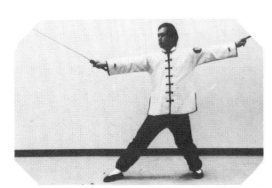

Fig.49

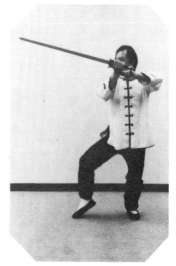

Fig.50

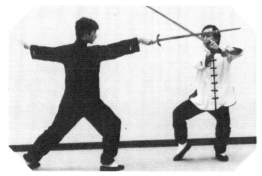

Fig.50A

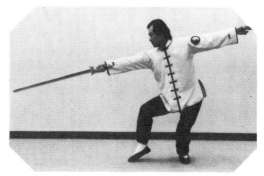

Fig.51

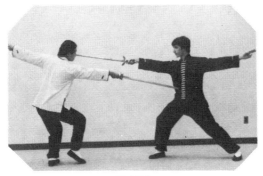

Fig.51A

165

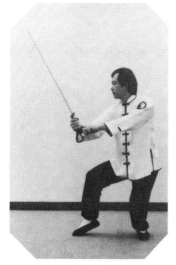

Fig.52

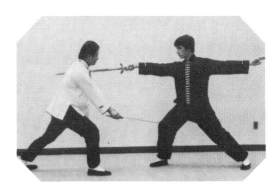

Fig.52A

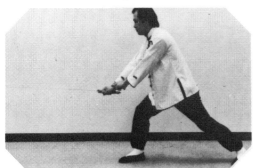

Fig.53

Fig.53A

18. Open Grass In Search of Snake (Poa Ts'ao Shoon Sir)

Figure 52: (W) Raise the sword up so that the flat part of the blade faces the front of the body. Inhale.

Figure 52A: The defender uses the lower part of the sword to guide an attack away.

Figure 53: (W) Shift onto your right leg so the stance is Deng San Bu. As the weight shifts, slide the sword forward at a level slightly above the knees. Exhale.

Figure 53A: The defender slices the opponent's knee after blocking.

Figure 54: (W) Lift your left leg and step slightly off to the left side. At the same time as the step, slide the sword forward about knee level. Your left hand is extended up. Inhale and exhale.

Figure 54A: The defender pushes an attack away and slices the opponent's knee.

Figure 55: (W) Lift your right leg and step slightly off to the right side. At the same time that your right leg steps off to the side, slide the sword forward near knee level. Inhale and exhale.

19. Hold the Moon Against the Chest (Fuai Chung Pao Yueh)

Figure 56: (W) Draw your right leg back so the stance is Shuen Gi Bu while turning and raising the sword up. Inhale.

20. Send the Bird to the Woods (Song Niao Shang Lin)

Figure 57: (W) Stand on your right leg and lift your left knee. Spread the arms open in an upward direction. Exhale.

Figure 57A: The defender attacks the neck with an upward motion of the sword.

166

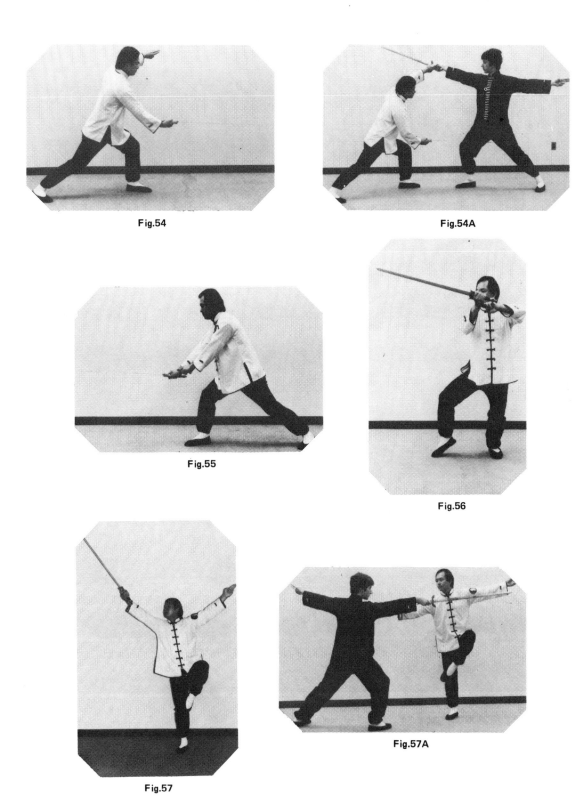

Fig.54

Fig.54A

Fig.55

Fig.56

Fig.57

Fig.57A

167

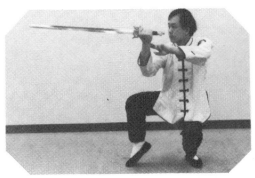

Fig.58

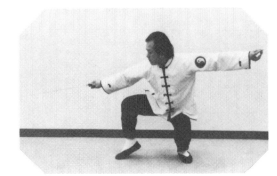

Fig.59

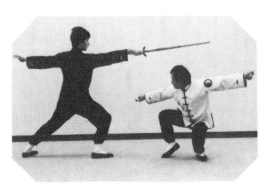

Fig.59A

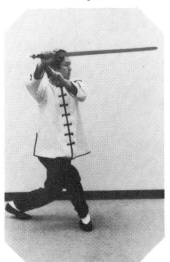

Fig.60

21. Black Dragon Waves Its Tail (Wu Long Bai Wei)

Figure 58: (W) Set your left leg down and draw your right leg up so the stance is Shuen Gi Bu, thigh parallel to the ground. At the same time, bring the sword down so it points W. Inhale.

Figure 59: (W) Slide the sword forward; the right palm faces down and the left hand extends back. Exhale.

Figure 59A: After blocking (Figure 58) the defender cuts the opponent's leg. This form may also be used to dodge a high attack while ducking low to counterattack.

22. Wind Blows the Lotus Leaf (Fong Chuan Ho Yeh)

Figure 60: (W) Set and turn your right leg so the stance is Dsao Pan Bu while moving the sword up, blade facing forward. Inhale.

Figure 60A: The defender turns and guides away a high attack.

Figure 61: (W) Step with your left leg forward into Deng San Bu while sliding the sword up. Exhale.

Figure 61A: The defender steps in to attack the neck of the opponent after guiding the sword away.

Figure 62: (W) Move the sword inward to the left side. The left hand touches the right wrist. Inhale.

Figure 62A: As the opponent attacks, the defender guides the attack away with the bottom edge of his sword.

Figure 63: (W) Push the sword out, right palm facing down. Exhale.

Figure 63A: After blocking, the defender slashes the neck of the opponent.

23. Lion Shakes Its Head (Shih Tzu Yao T'ou)

Figure 64: (E) Turn your body 180 degrees clockwise while swinging the sword across the body. Inhale.

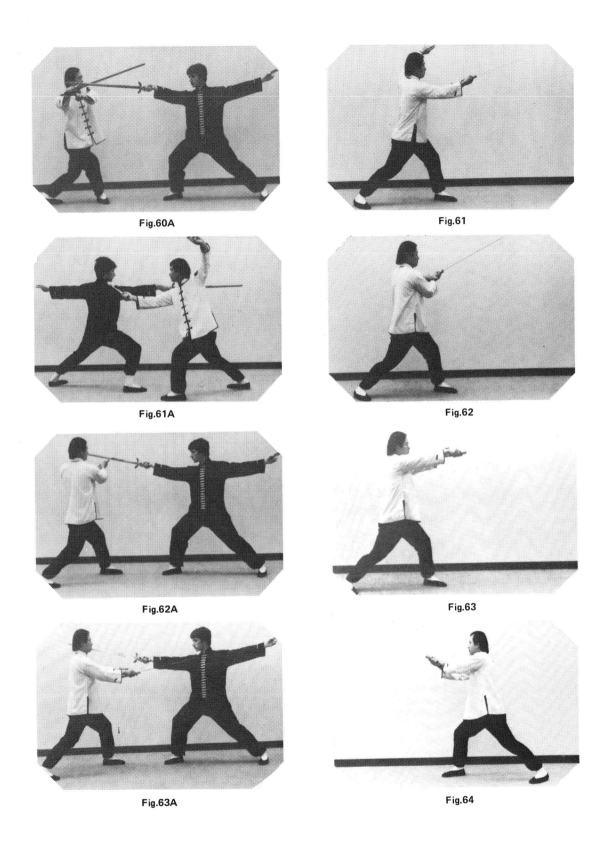

Fig.60A

Fig.61

Fig.61A

Fig.62

Fig.62A

Fig.63

Fig.63A

Fig.64

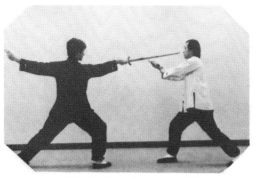

Fig.64A

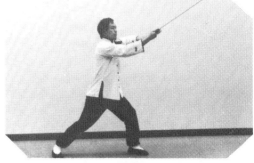

Fig.65

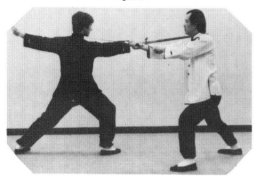

Fig.65A

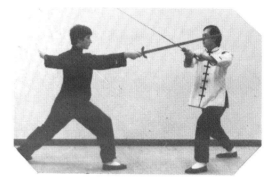

Fig.65B

Figure 64A: When an opponent stabs, the defender pushes the attacker's sword to the side with the lower edge of his sword.

Figure 65: (E) Step your left leg forward and to the side. Move your right leg slightly to the left so that the stance is Deng San Bu. While in the process of moving the body, slash the sword across the front of your body by using only the wrists to accomplish this motion. Exhale.

Figure 65A: After blocking, the defender steps to the side and slashes the opponent's throat with the sword by using a whipping action created by the wrists.

Figure 65B: When Figure 65 is finished, it also begins another block, but from an inside position.

Figure 66: (E) Step your right leg forward and to the side. Move your left leg slightly to the right; feet are thus aligned in Deng San Bu. While moving, slash the sword across your body by using only the wrists. Inhale.

Figure 66A: Once the opponent's sword is neutralized, the defender slashes the attacker's throat.

Figure 67: (E) Repeat Figure 65. Inhale.

Figure 68: (E) Repeat Figure 66. Exhale.

24. Tiger Holds Its Head (Fu Pao T'ou)

Figure 69: (E) Draw the sword in and shift the stance to Shuen Gi Bu. Inhale.

25. Wild Horse Jumps the Stream (Yeh Ma T'iao Jen)

Figure 70: (E) Jump off the right leg and repeat Figure 29. Exhale.

Figure 71: (E) Repeat Figure 30. Complete exhalation.

26. Turn Body and Rein In Horse (Fan Shen Duh Ma)

Figure 72: (W) Turn your body 180 degrees counterclockwise into Deng San Bu, left leg forward, while swinging your left hand across your body. Inhale.

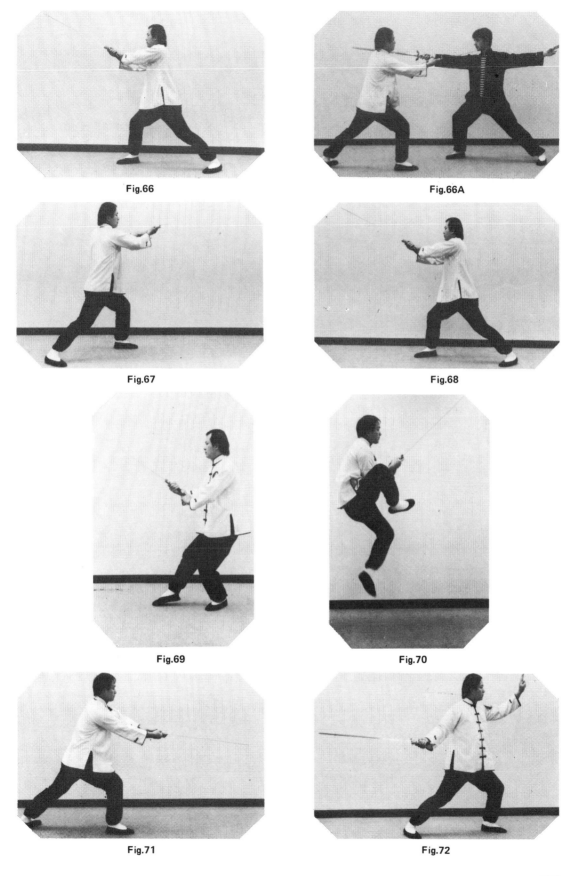

Fig.66

Fig.66A

Fig.67

Fig.68

Fig.69

Fig.70

Fig.71

Fig.72

171

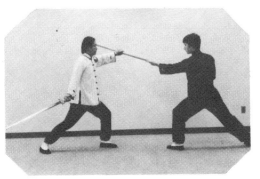

Fig.72A

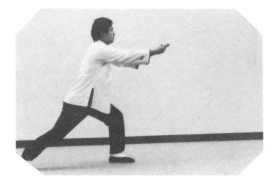

Fig.73

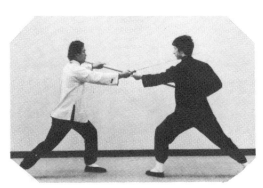

Fig.73A

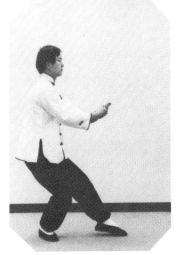

Fig.74

Figure 72A: As an opponent attacks with a rod, the defender pushes it to the side.

Figure 73: (W) Swing the sword all the way around to the left hand. Begin exhalation.

Figure 73A: After blocking the rod, the defender cuts the attacker's neck.

Figure 74: (W) Draw in the sword and shift stance to Shuen Gi Bu. Continue exhalation.

Figure 74A: After cutting the neck, the defender slides his sword over the opponent's wrist.

27. Compass (Chih Nan Chen)

Figure 75: (W) Bring your right leg up and push the sword slightly up while squatting. Complete exhalation.

Figure 75A: Once the wrists have been cut, the defender moves in to stab the chest or neck area.

28. Clean Up Dust In the Wind (Ying Fong Tan Ch'en)

Figure 76: (W) Left your right knee up and turn the sword up, right palm facing the side. Inhale.

Figure 76A: The defender blocks an attack with the lower edge of his sword.

Figure 77: (NW) Move your right leg NW into Deng San Bu while pushing the sword forward from your chest. Exhale.

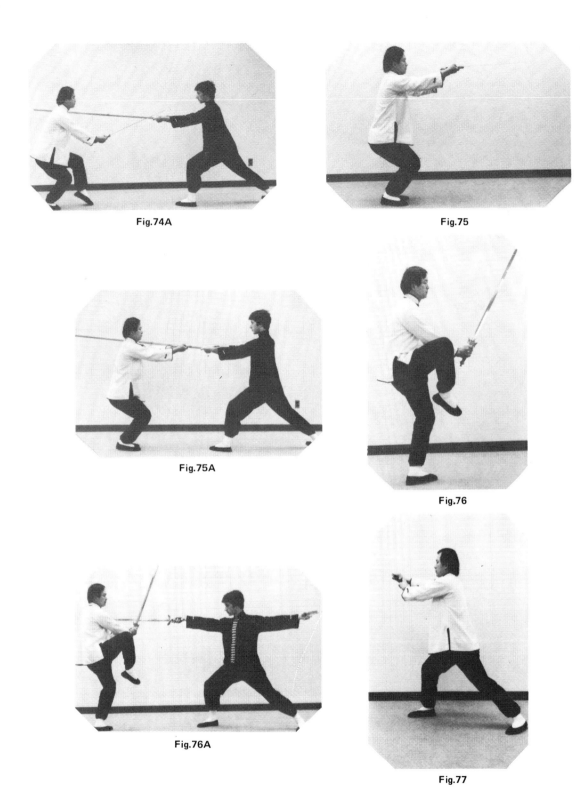

Fig.74A

Fig.75

Fig.75A

Fig.76

Fig.76A

Fig.77

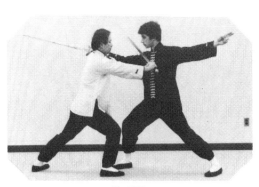

Fig.77A

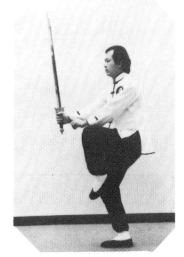

Fig.78

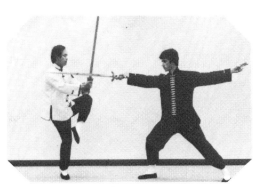

Fig.78A

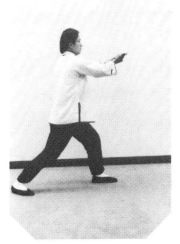

Fig.79

Figure 77A: Once the block is complete, the defender slides in and strikes the opponent with the lower edge of the sword. The defender thus hits, rather than cuts, the opponent.

Figure 78: (NW) Lift your left knee and turn the sword up. The right palm faces the side. Inhale.

Figure 78A: The defender blocks an attack from an outside position.

Figure 79: (SW) Move your left leg to the SW and push the sword forward from your chest. The stance is Deng San Bu.

Figure 79A: After the block, the defender attacks the opponent's neck with the lower edge of the sword.

Figure 80: (SW) Lift your right knee up and turn the sword up, right palm pointed to the side. Inhale.

Figure 81: (NW) Repeat Figure 77. Exhale.

29. Push Boat With the Current (Shun Shui T'uai Chou)

Figure 82: (W) Move your right leg to the left side so it crosses your left leg. At the same time, slide the sword down to where the right leg is positioned. Inhale.

Figure 82A: The defender slides away an attack to his lower body.

Figure 83: (W) Step forward with your left leg into Deng San Bu while swinging the sword back, up, forward, and down. The left hand releases itself from the right wrist and retouches the wrist when the sword is overhead. Exhale.

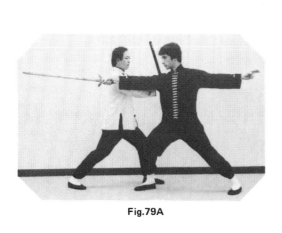

Fig.79A

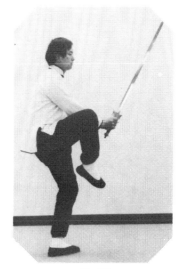

Fig.80

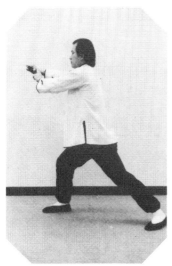

Fig.81

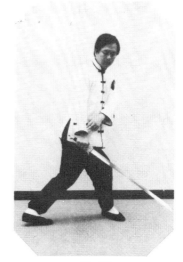

Fig.82

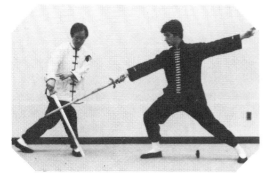

Fig.82A

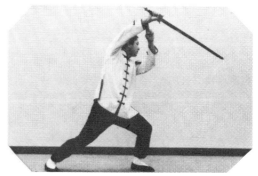

Fig.83

175

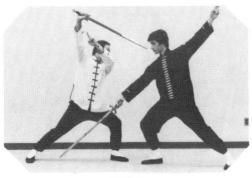

Fig.83A

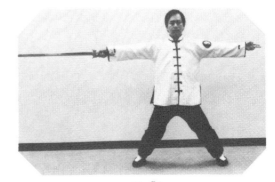

Fig.84

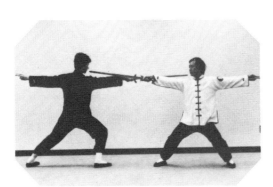

Fig.84A

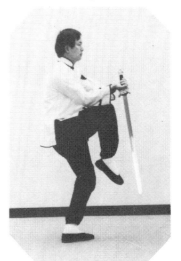

Fig.85

Figure 83A: Once the low attack is guided away, the defender steps in to stab the opponent from the top.

30. Shooting Star Chasing the Moon (Lieo Hsing Kan Yeuh)

Figure 84: (N) Change the stance into Ma Bu and swing the sword over the head and down to shoulder level. The sword points E. Inhale.

Figure 84A: The defender dodges an attack and then cuts the hand of the opponent.

31. Bird Flying Over the Waterfall (T'ien Niao Fei P'u)

Figure 85: (N) Raise your right knee and let the sword fall back. Inhale.

Figure 85A: The defender slides a low attack away.

Figure 86: (N) Step forward with your right leg and place both feet together while swinging the sword up and then down. Exhale.

Figure 86A: The defender slides the sword down on the opponent's head after the block.

33. Raise the Screen (T'iao Lien Shih)

Figure 87: (E) Bring your right leg back so that the front of your body faces E. While moving back, slide the sword up so it is horizontal to the ground. Inhale.

Figure 87A: The defender slides away a high attack.

Figure 88: (E) Raise your left foot on its toe while swinging the sword down and up to the left side. Exhale.

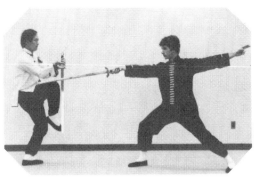

Fig.85A

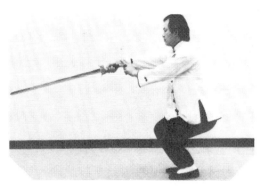

Fig.86

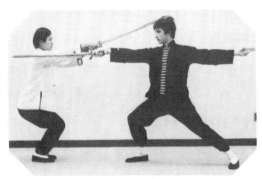

Fig.86A

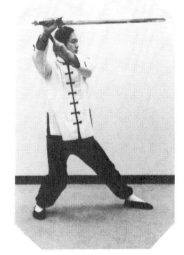

Fig.87

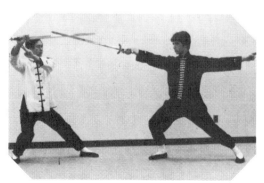

Fig.87A

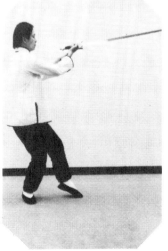

Fig.88

177

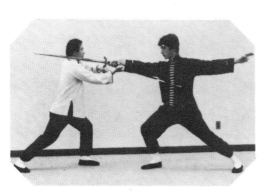

Fig.88A

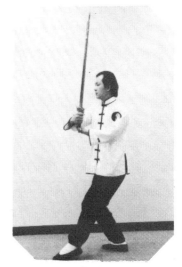

Fig.89

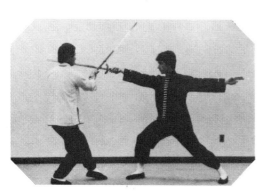

Fig.89A

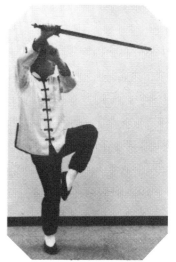

Fig.90

Figure 88A: After blocking, the defender slides under the attack and up into the opponent's abdomen.

Figure 89: (E) Continue to swing the sword up, but turn right palm so the sword is perpendicular to the ground. Inhale.

Figure 89A: As the defender's sword moves up, he slides away an attack to the side.

Figure 90: (E) Swing the sword back, down, and up to the right side while lifting your left knee. Exhale.

Figure 90A: The defender slides under the attack to slash the opponent.

33. Left and Right Wheel Sword (Tso Yu Ch'e Lun Chien)

Figure 91: (E) Step down with your left leg and turn it out so that the stance is Dsao Pan Bu. At the same time, swing the sword down and back. The left hand touches the right wrist. Inhale.

Figure 91A: The defender slides a low attack away.

Figure 92: (E) Bring your right leg forward and slide the sword up and straight ahead. The right palm faces the body and the left hand points back. Exhale.

Figure 92A: The defender slides the sword up to stab the opponent in the neck.

Figure 93: (E) Turn your right leg so the stance is Dsao Pan Bu and slide the sword down and back while spinning the blade. The right palm turns in. Inhale.

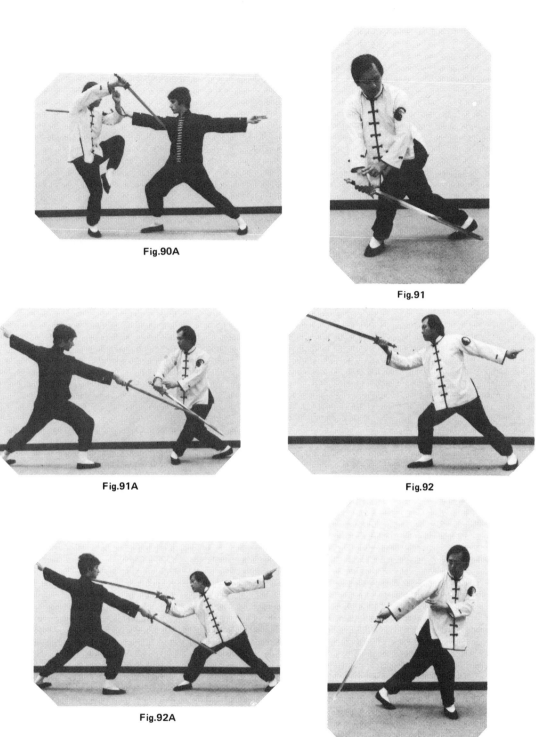

Fig.90A

Fig.91

Fig.91A

Fig.92

Fig.92A

Fig.93

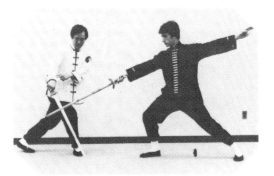

Fig.93A

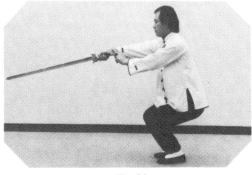

Fig.94

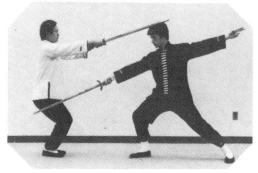

Fig.94A

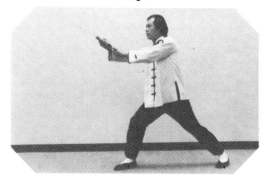

Fig.95

Figure 93A: As the opponent lunges for the legs, the defender guides away the attack.

34. Swallow Picks Up Mud With Beak (Yen Tzu Shen Ni)

Figure 94: (E) Swing the sword back, up, and forward while stepping straight ahead with your left leg. Next, bring your right leg forward so both legs are together. Squat slightly. Exhale.

Figure 94A: After blocking in Figure 93, the defender steps forward to counterattack over the top.

35. A Roc Spreads Its Wings (Ta P'eng Chan Ch'ih)

Figure 95: (W) Move your right leg back and turn the body 180 degrees clockwise. Swing the sword up while keeping your left hand on the right wrist. The stance is Deng San Bu. Inhale and exhale.

Figure 95A: The defender dodges an attack and then cuts the opponent's wrist.

36. Pick Up the Moon From the Sea Bottom (Hai Ti Lao Yueh)

Figure 96: (E) Turn the body 180 degrees counterclockwise while swinging your left hand in front of your face. The sword stays behind. Inhale.

Figure 96A: The left hand pushes a rod attack to the side.

Figure 97: (E) Move your right leg forward into Deng San Bu and swing the sword down at knee level; your upper body leans forward. The left hand extends up and back. Exhale.

Figure 97A: This is a long range attack by the defender. After pushing the rod away, he leans forward to cut the opponent's knee.

37. Hold the Moon Against the Chest (Fuai Chung Pao Yueh)

Figure 98: (N) Repeat Figure 56. Inhale. The sword points W.

Figure 98A: The defender slides away an attack to his face by the lower edge of his sword.

38. Night Demon Gauges the Depth of the Sea (Yeh Ch'a T'an Hai)

Figure 99: (N) Raise your left knee and stab toward N. The blade points down and your left hand extends back. Exhale.

180

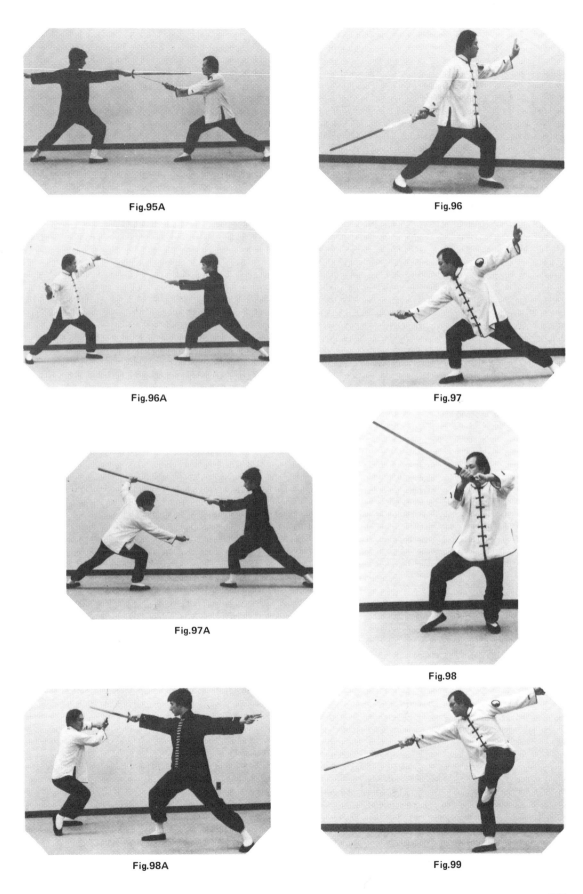

Fig.95A

Fig.96

Fig.96A

Fig.97

Fig.97A

Fig.98

Fig.98A

Fig.99

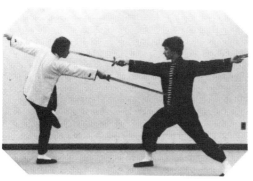

Fig.99A

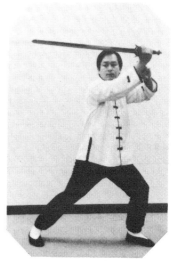

Fig.100

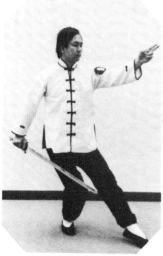

Fig.101

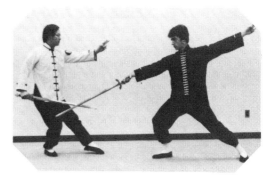

Fig.101A

Figure 99A: After sliding the attack away, the defender moves his sword staight in to the stomach.

39. A Rhino Looks at the Moon (Hsi Nieu Wang Yueh)

Figure 100: (N) Move your left leg down to W and slide the sword up, right palm facing in. Begin to inhale.

40. Shoot the Geese (Sheh Yen Shih)

Figure 101: (W) Turn your body to the W while shifting the stance to Shuen Gi Bu, sliding the sword down past your right hip. As the sword moves down, extend your left hand. Complete inhalation.

Figure 101A: The defender slides away a low attack with the flat part of the sword.

41. Blue Dragon Waves His Claws (Ch'ing Long T'an Jwa)

Figure 102: (W) Move your right leg to your left leg and extend the sword forward. Squat slightly. Exhale.

Figure 102A: After sliding the low attack away, the defender moves in to stab the opponent in the side.

42. Phoenix Spreads Its Wings (Fong Huang Shuang Chan Ch'ih)

Figure 103: (E) Turn your body 180 degrees clockwise and repeat Figures 38 and 39. Inhale and exhale.

43. Left and Right Step Over Obstacle (Tso Yu K'ua Lan)

Figure 104: (E) Raise the sword straight up and left the left knee. Inhale.

Figure 104A: The defender uses the lower part of the sword to guide an attack away from the outside position.

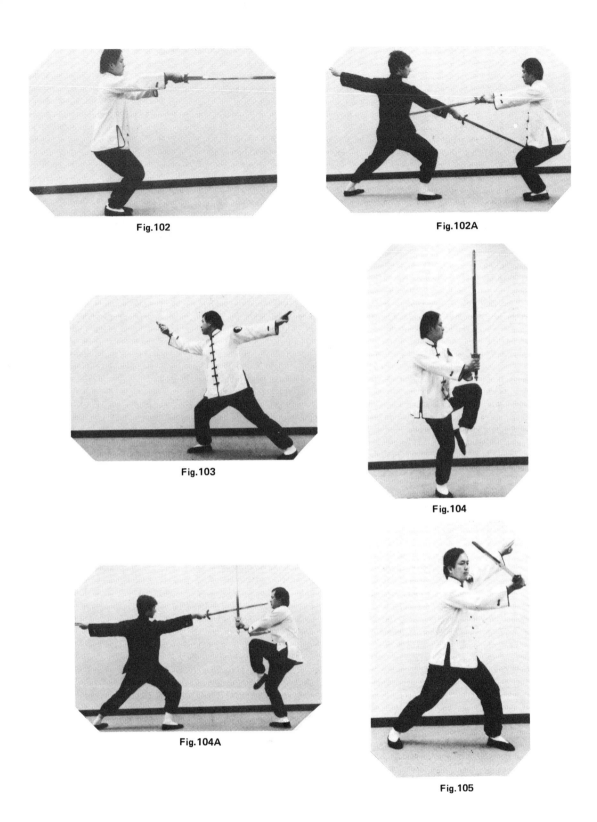

Fig.102

Fig.102A

Fig.103

Fig.104

Fig.104A

Fig.105

Figure 105: (NE) Move your left leg NE and slide the sword forward at about neck level. The sword is perpendicular to the body. Exhale.

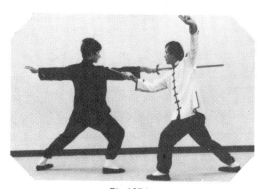

Fig.105A

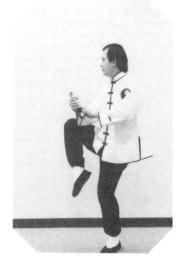

Fig.106

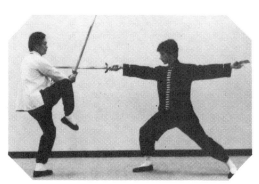

Fig.106A

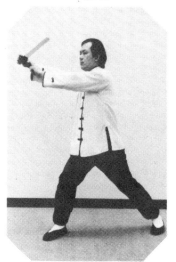

Fig.107

Figure 105A: After blocking, the defender moves in over the top of the opponent's arm to slash the neck.

Figure 106: (E) Raise the sword, right palm facing in, and lift your right knee. Inhale.

Figure 106A: The defender slides away an attack from the inside position.

Figure 107: (SE) Move your right leg to the SE and slide the sword forward at about neck level. Exhale.

Figure 107A: The defender slashes the opponent's neck after blocking.

44. Shoot the Geese (Sheh Yen Shih)

Figure 108: (E) Slide the sword down past your right hip while bringing your left leg forward so the stance is Shuen Gi Bu. As the sword moves down, extend your left hand. Inhale.

45. White Ape Offers Up Fruit (Pai Yuen Hsien Guoo)

Figure 109: (E) Repeat Figure 102. Exhale.

46. Falling Flowers Posture (Loa Fua Shih)

Figure 110: (E) Move your right leg back and circle the sword down and up to your left side. The left hand touches the right wrist. Inhale.

Figure 110A: As the opponent attacks high, the defender guides the sword away, using the lower edge of his sword.

Figure 111: (E) Swing the sword so that the tip moves up, back, down, then up and forward; the sword ends its motion on the upper right side of the practitioner's body. Exhale.

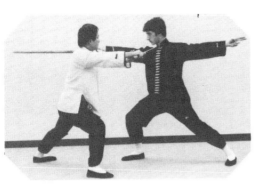

Fig.107A

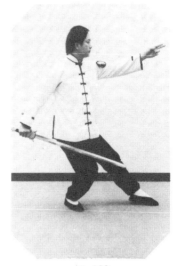

Fig.108

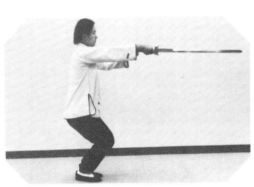

Fig.109

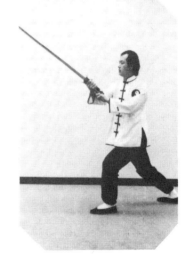

Fig.110

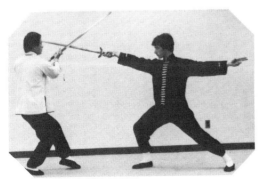

Fig.110A

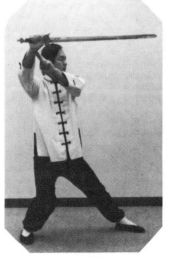

Fig.111

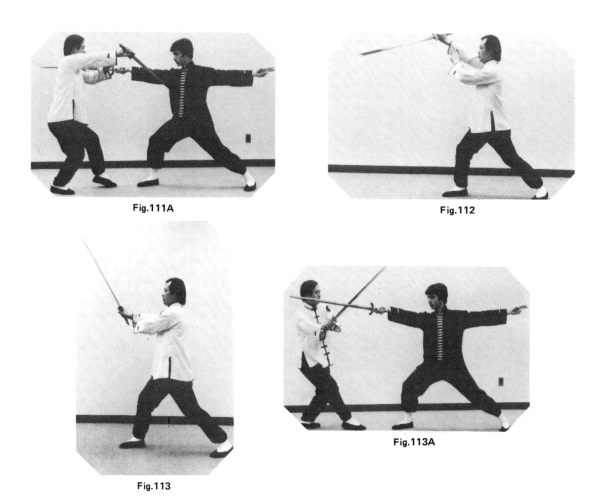

Fig.111A

Fig.112

Fig.113

Fig.113A

Figure 111A: The defnder counterattacks by sliding his sword underneath the opponent's weapon so that the armpit is cut.

Figure 112: (E) Move your left leg back. Raise your right hand higher than the sword. Begin to inhale.

Figure 113: (E) Swing the sword up while keeping your right hand relatively stable. Complete inhalation.

Figure 113A: The defender blocks from an outside position.

Figure 114: (E) Move your right leg back while swinging the sword so its tip circles up, back, then up and forward to the left side. Exhale.

Figure 114A: After blocking, counterattack by sliding the sword underneath the opponent's weapon.

47. Fair Lady Weaves Shuttle (Yu Nu Ch'uan Suo)

Figure 115: (S) Raise your left knee and turn your head and the side of your body to S. Swing the sword so that the blade points N. Inhale.

Figure 115A: The defender slides away an attack to the chest.

Figure 116: (S) Swing the sword up and then down until the blade is horizontal. Exhale.

Figure 116A: The defender attacks over the top once the block is complete.

Figure 117: (N) Set your left leg down and turn N. Turn the sword in so that the blade points N. Inhale.

Figure 118: (N) Shift the stance to Deng San Bu and push the sword forward and down. Exhale.

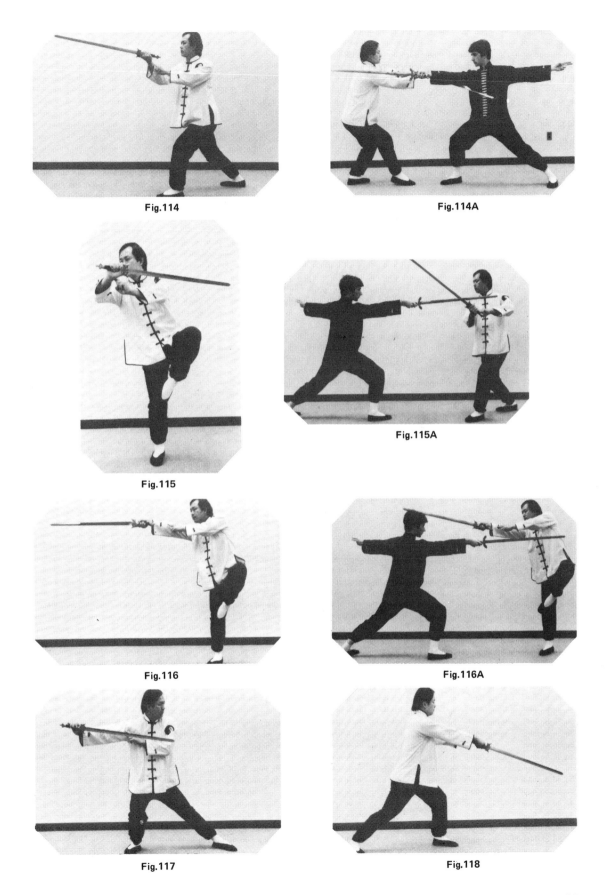

Fig.114

Fig.114A

Fig.115

Fig.115A

Fig.116

Fig.116A

Fig.117

Fig.118

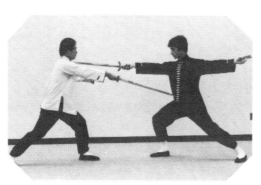

Fig.118A

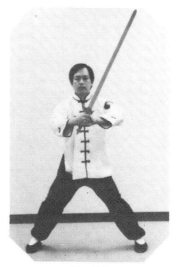

Fig.119

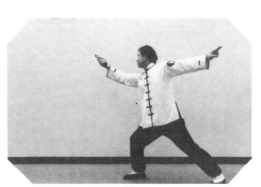

Fig.120

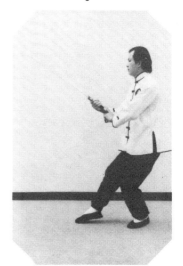

Fig. 121

Figure 118A: The defender dodges an attack and stabs down.

48. White Tiger Waves Its Tail (Pai Fu Chow Wei)
Figure 119: (E) Turn your body 90 degrees clockwise and repeat Figure 38. Begin to inhale.

Figure 120: (S) Turn another 90 degrees and repeat Figure 39. Complete inhalation.

49. Fish Jumps Into Dragon Gate (Yu T'iao Long Mun)
Figure 121: (E) Turn your body E and repeat Figure 69. Exhale.

Figure 122: (E) Repeat Figure 29. Inhale.

Figure 123: (E) Repeat Figure 30. Exhale.

50. Black Dragon Wraps Around Post (Wu Long Chow Tsuh)
Figure 124: (E) Step forward with your left leg and repeat Figure 24. Inhale.

Figure 125: (E) Repeat Figure 25. Begin to exhale.

Figure 126: (SW) Turn your body 135 degrees clockwise while shifting the stance to Deng San Bu, right leg forward, and swinging the sword straight down until it is a little past the shoulder. Complete exhalation.

Figure 126A: The defender dodges an attack and cuts the opponent's wrist.

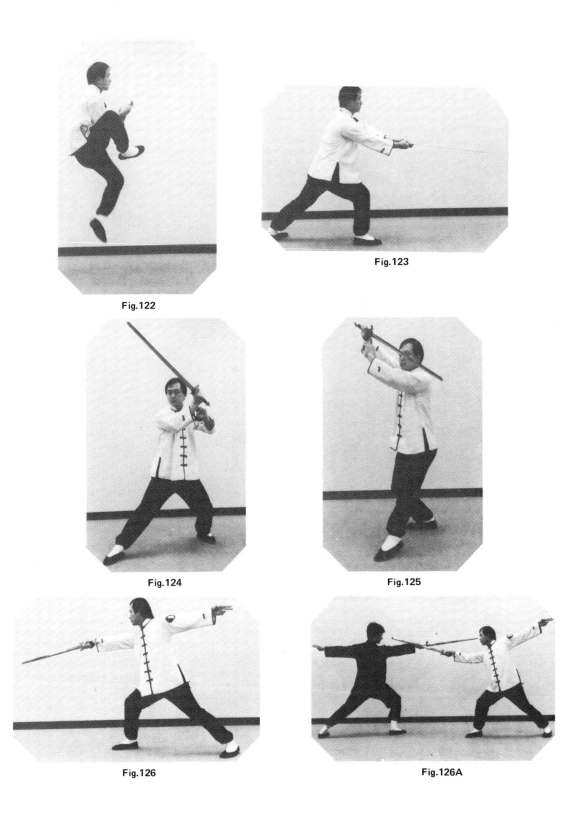

Fig.122

Fig.123

Fig.124

Fig.125

Fig.126

Fig.126A

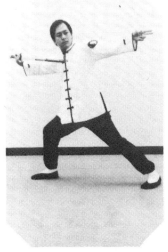

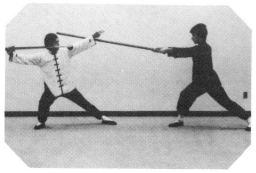

Fig.127A

Fig.127

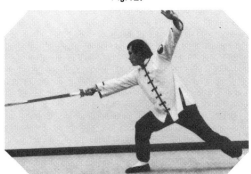

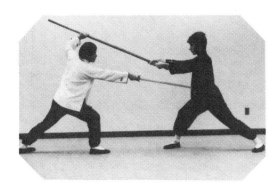

Fig.128

Fig.128A

Figure 127: (SW) Turn the sword in; face looks E. Inhale.

Figure 127A: As an opponent attacks with a rod, the defender slides the weapon away with the left hand.

Figure 128: (E) Step forward with your right leg and push the sword forward and down. Exhale.

Figure 128A: After pushing the rod away, the defender moves in to stab the opponent.

51. Fairy Shows the Way: Second Form (Hsien Jen Chih Lu)

Figure 129: (E) Sit back in Ssu Lieu Bu and slide the sword back to the left side. Your right palm faces in and your left hand touches right wrist. Inhale.

Figure 129A: The defender pushes an attack away.

Figure 130: (E) Shift the stance to Deng San Bu while sliding the sword forward. Exhale.

Figure 130A: After blocking, the defender moves in to cut the opponent's neck.

52. Wind Blows Away the Plum Flowers (Fong Sao Mei Hua)

Figure 131: (N) Spin 360 degrees clockwise on your right leg while extending both arms straight out. Begin to inhale.

Figure 132: (N) Set your left leg down while moving the sword up. Complete inhalation.

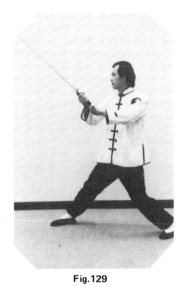

Fig.129

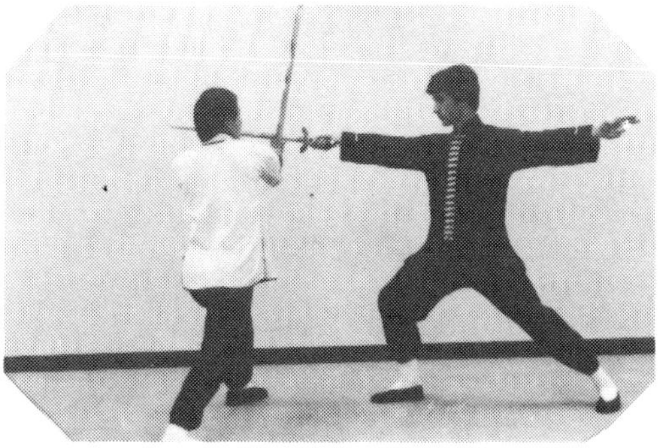

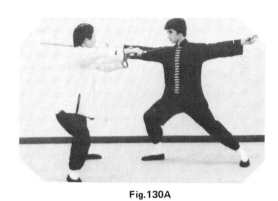

Fig.129A

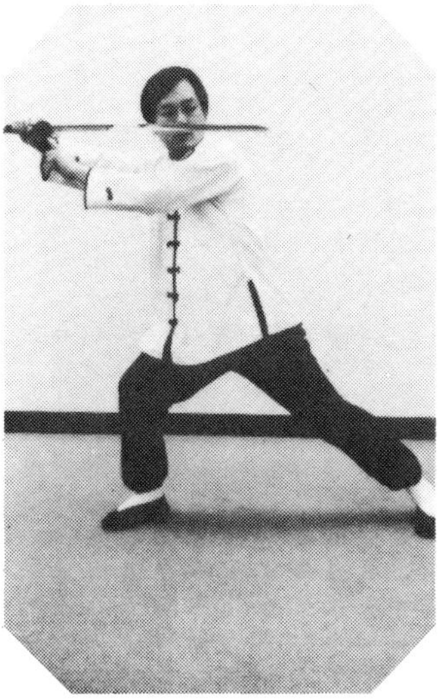

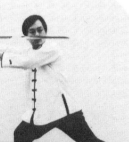

Fig.130

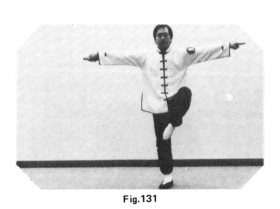

Fig.130A

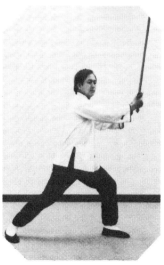

Fig.131

Fig.132

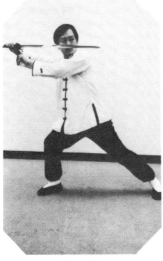

Fig.133

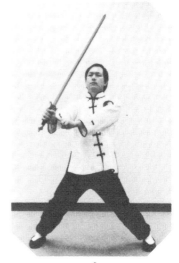

Fig.134

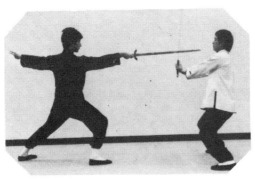

Fig.134A

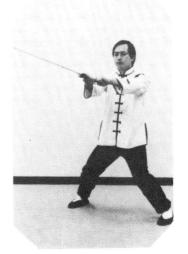

Fig.135

Figure 133: (N) Shift the stance to Deng San Bu, right leg forward, while sliding the sword toward the front of the body. Exhale.

53. To Hold A Tablet (Shou P'eng Ya Fu)

Figure 134: (N) Switch the stance to Ma Bu while circling the sword clockwise in front of your body. Your head leans back. Inhale.

Figure 134A: The defender guides an attack to the face off to the side.

Figure 135: (N) Move your left leg and then your right leg forward into Ma Bu while sliding the sword forward. Exhale.

Figure 135A: After blocking, the defender moves in to stab the opponent in the neck.

54. Hold the Sword and Return to the Original Stance (Pao Jen Kuai Yuan)

Figure 136: (N) Move the sword back and down while your left hand cups your right. Begin to inhale.

Figure 137: (N) The sword then moves back, up, and forward while it is switched to your left hand. Your left hand grabs the sword as in the very beginning of the sequence. Complete inhalation.

Figure 138: (N) Your left hand swings down while your right hand moves down and up. Begin exhalation.

Figure 139: (N) Your right hand moves down to end the sequence. Complete exhalation.

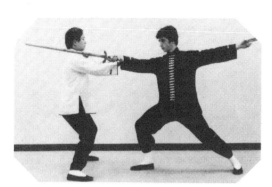

Fig.135A

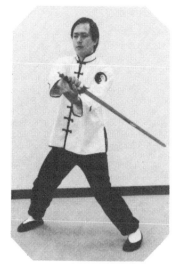

Fig.136

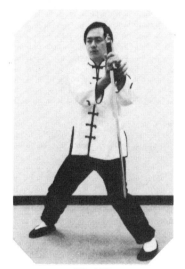

Fig.137

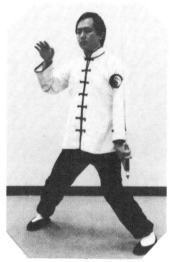

Fig.138

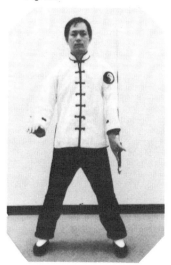

Fig.139

Tai Chi Narrow Blade Sword Fighting Forms

Before starting the narrow blade fighting forms, the student should review their purpose as it was stated in the beginning of this chapter. For ease of reference, the martial artist in the white top shall be referred to as W, while the martial artist in the black top shall be referred to as B.

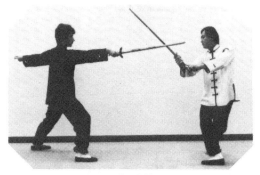

Fig. 140

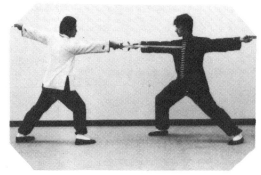

Fig. 141

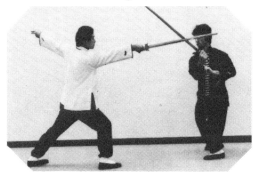

Fig. 142

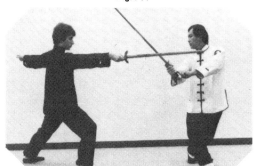

Fig. 143

Fighting Form 1

Figure 140: B stabs at W. W uses the lower part of the blade to slide the attack away. While W is sliding the attack away, he moves to the side by crossing his left leg behind his right.

Figure 141: W steps forward, uncrossing his legs, and stabs at B.

Figure 142: B counters by sliding the stab away in the same manner as W while moving to the side by crossing his legs. B then steps the lead leg forward and stabs at W. Next, W begins the cycle over by blocking again.

Fighting Form 2

Figure 143: B stabs at W. W slides the attack away while stepping to the side by crossing his legs.

Figure 144: W steps to the side with his front leg and stabs a B's temple area.

Figure 145: B crosses his legs and slides the attack away.

Figure 146: B steps to the side with his front leg and stabs at W's temple. W counters by stepping to the side, crossing his legs, then uncrossing his legs and stepping to the side, stabbing at B's temple.

Fighting Form 3

Figure 147: B cuts at W with a horizontal slash. W dodges the attack by moving to the side by crossing his legs, using the sword to slide the attack away.

Figure 148: W steps to the side with the front leg and cuts at B's neck.

Figure 149: B slides the attack to the side while crossing his legs to dodge the maneuver.

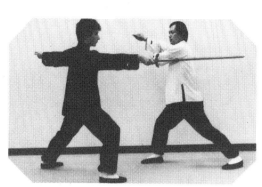

Fig.144

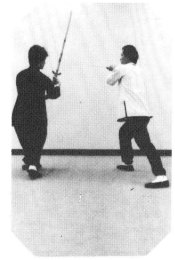

Fig.145

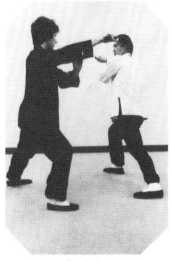

Fig.146

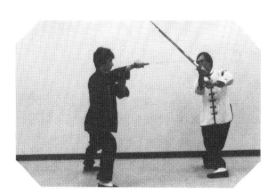

Fig.147

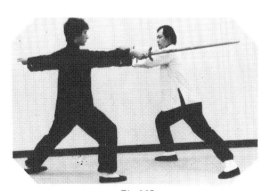

Fig.148

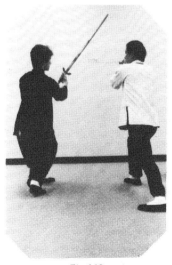

Fig.149

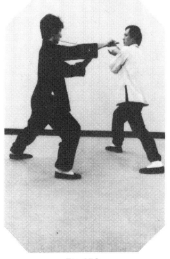

Fig.150

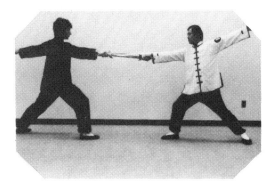

Fig.151

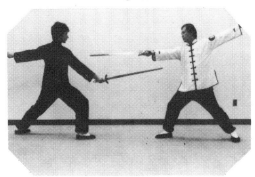

Fig.152

Fig.153

Figure 150: B steps to the side with the front leg while cutting at W's neck. W counters as in Figure 147 to begin the cycle again.

Fighting Form 4

Figure 151: B stabs low at W. W circles his sword up to cut B's wrist while avoiding B's attack.

Figure 152: To avoid getting his wrist cut, B moves his wrist down while keeping the tip of his sword stationary.

Figure 153: B circles his sword up to cut W on the wrist.

Figure 154: To avoid getting cut, W moves his wrist down while keeping the tip of his sword stationary.

Figure 155: W then circles his weapon around B's sword in order to cut B's wrist. In total, both practitioners are circling their wrists up and down while the tip of their swords remain at one point. This fighting form is specialized training for attacking the opponent's wrist.

Fighting Form 5

Figure 156: B stabs at W. W avoids the attack by crossing his left leg in back of his right leg. W does not use his sword to slide the attack away; he merely dodges.

Figure 157: W steps with his front leg to the side and cuts down on B's wrist.

Figure 158: B avoids W's attack by stepping to the side, crossing his legs. At the same time that B is moving, he drops his sword hand down and in.

Figure 159: B steps to the side with his front leg and cuts down on W's wrist. W counters by duplicating his original movement.

Fighting Form 6

Figure 160: B stabs at W. W crosses his right leg in front of his left and cuts down on B's wrist.

Figure 161: To counter, B crosses his legs in the same manner as W while cutting down on W's wrist. This fighting form is the mirror of the previous one.

196

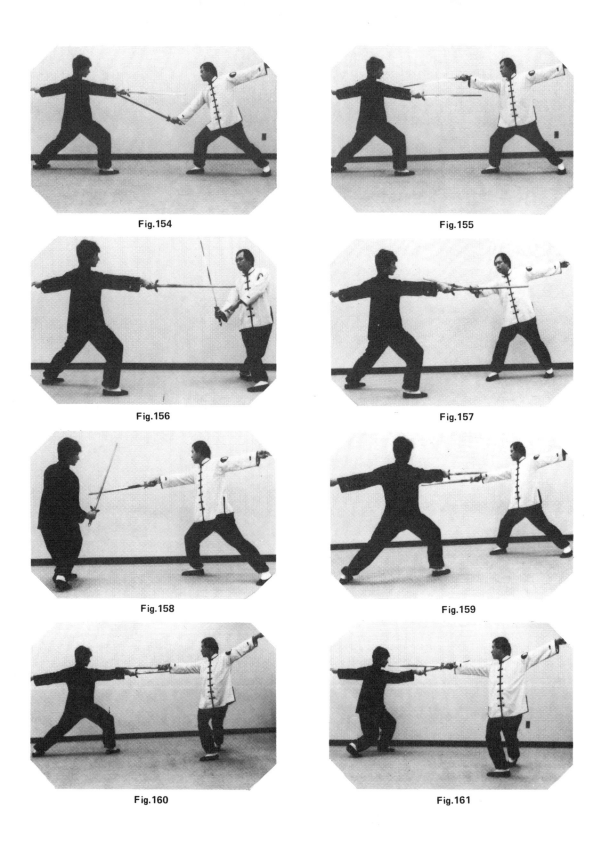

Fig.154

Fig.155

Fig.156

Fig.157

Fig.158

Fig.159

Fig.160

Fig.161

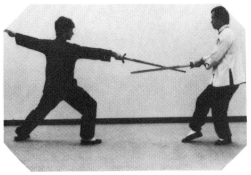

Fig.162

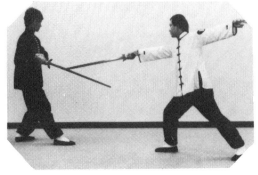

Fig.163

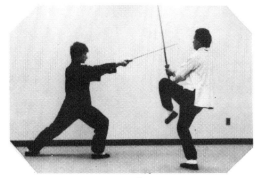

Fig.164

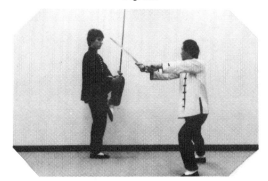

Fig.165

Fighting Form 7

Figure 162: B stabs at W's abdomen. W slides his sword down to guide the attack away.

Figure 163: After blocking, W stabs down at B's abdomen. B then slides his sword back to dissolve W's attack. B stabs at W to renew the cycle.

Fighting Form 8

Figure 164: B cuts at W's neck. W swings his sword from underneath and slides the attack away to the side. At the same time that W dissolves B's attack, he lifts his outside knee.

Figure 165: W sets his leg down to the side and cuts at B's neck from the outside. B then slides his sword up and guides W's attack away while raising his outside knee. B then steps down to the side and cuts at W's neck to start the cycle.

Fighting Form 9

Figure 166: B slashes at W' neck in a clockwise swing. W leans his head back and uses a clockwise sweep of the sword to guide the attack away.

Figure 167: W continues his circle and in his turn slashes at B's neck. B slides his sword clockwise to guide W's sword away. B in his turn continues the sweep of his sword so he once again attacks W's neck.

Fighting Form 10

Figure 168: B attacks W's neck by sweeping his sword in a counterclockwise motion. W slides his sword up counterclockwise to guide the attack away from the side.

Figure 169: W then slashes forward at B's neck. B slides his sword back counterclockwise to neutralize W's attack. B then slashes forward to begin the cycle.

Fighting Form 11

Figure 170: Both practitioners stand with their left legs forward and their swords across the body.

Figure 171: Both practitioners jump off their left leg while cutting down at each other's wrist. Each keeps jumping off the left leg in a circle once their right legs have touched down. Each time they jump they must cut down on the other's wrist.

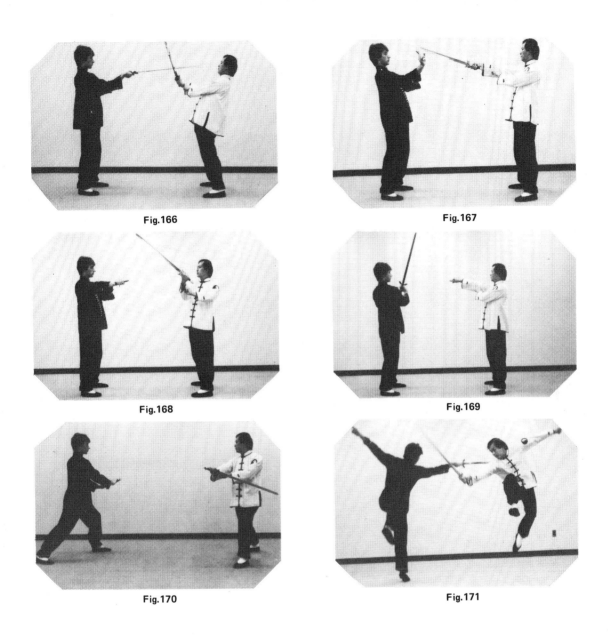

Fig.166

Fig.167

Fig.168

Fig.169

Fig.170

Fig.171

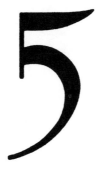

CONCLUSION

The author hopes that this volume has succeeded in presenting the martial and exercise aspects of Tai Chi Chuan for both the martial artist and the individual interested in health. To achieve either aspect will require patience on the part of the practitioner. Unlike may other systems of martial training as well as other sports, the person taking up Tai Chi must develop an inner calm that only can grow out of a patient and perservering mind. In essence, the mind of the individual is the key to success of Tai Chi Chuan.

Because Tai Chi requires a developed mind, when anybody begins the study of Tai Chi, it will take time for positive results to be seen. But once the individual has developed enough patience to practice Tai Chi consistently and seriously, the benefits will be many. To achieve good health or martial power through Tai Chi, the practitioner must be willing to sacrifice some time each day; but in the end, the person will gain more than the initial sacrifice because of improved health and a sound mind.

In this day and age, the aspects of mind which Tai Chi develops are much needed. As the fast-paced modern world accelerates its pressures and demands, more people will be forced to find a quiet center of peace to avoid breaking down. Because Tai Chi demands no more than a few feet of space to practice, it can offer the modern, pressure-packed world a serene haven which will freshen the body and renew the spirit.

In terms of the skills presented in this book, almost the whole range of Tai Chi Chuan is shown to the student. With such a book, the practitioner may at any time go on to other aspects which may interest him—anything from still meditation to the Tai Chi narrow blade sword. In addition, with the foundation presented in this book, the student may use it as a base for his own further research and practice of aspects that are not covered in this book.

APPENDIX A

YANG'S TAI CHI CH'UAN (LARGE STYLE AND LOW POSTURE)

No.	Chinese	English	Pronunciation
1.	太極起勢	Beginning	T'ai-Chi-Ch'i Shih
2.	右攬雀尾	Grasp Sparrow's Tail: Right	Yu Lan Ch'iao Wei
3.	左攬雀尾	Grasp Sparrow's Tail: Left	Tso Lan Ch'iao Wei
4.	掤	Ward Off	P'eng
5.	攦	Rollback	Lu
6.	擠	Press	Ghi
7.	按	Push	An
8.	單鞭	Single Whip	Tan Pien
9.	提手上式	Lift Hands and Lean Forward	T'i Shou Shang Shih
10.	白鶴亮翅	The Crane Spreads Its Wings	Pai Hao Liang Ch'ih
11.	左摟膝拗步	Brush Knee and Step Forward: Left	Tso Lou Hsi Yao Pu
12.	手揮琵琶	Play the Guitar	Shou Hui P'i P'a
13.	左摟膝拗步	Brush Knee and Step Forward: Left	Tso Lou Hsi Yao Pu
14.	右摟膝拗步	Brush Knee and Step Forward: Right	Yu Lou Hsi Yao Pu
15.	左摟膝拗步	Brush Knee and Step Forward: Left	Tso Lou Hsi Yao Pu
16.	手揮琵琶	Play the Guitar	Shou Hui P'i P'a
17.	左摟膝拗步	Brush Knee and Step Forward: Left	Tso Lou Hsi Yao Pu
18.	撇身捶	Twist Body and Circle Fist	Pieh Shen Ch'ui
19.	進步搬攔捶	Step Forward, Deflect Downward, Parry and Punch	Chin Pu Pan Lan Ch'ui
20.	如封似閉	Seal Tightly	Ju Feng Ssu Pi
21.	抱虎歸山	Embrace Tiger and Return to the Mountain	Pao Hu Guei Shan
22.	合太極	Close Tai Chi	Ho T'ai-Chi
23.	掤攦擠按	Ward-Off, Rollback, Press and Push	Peng, Lu, Ghi, An
24.	單鞭	Single Whip	Tan Pien
25.	肘底看捶	Punch Under the Elbow	Chou Ti K'an Ch'ui
26.	左倒攆猴	Step Back and Repulse Monkey: Left	Tso Tao Nien Hou
27.	右倒攆猴	Step Back and Repulse Monkey: Right	Yu Tao Nien Hou
28.	左倒攆猴	Step Back and Repulse Monkey: Left	Tso Tao Nien Hou
29.	斜飛勢	Diagonal Flying	Hsieh Fei Shih
30.	提手上勢	Lift Hands and Lean Forward	T'i Shou Shang Shih
31.	白鶴亮翅	The Crane Spreads Its Wings	Pai Hao Liang Ch'ih
32.	左摟膝拗步	Brush Knee and Step Forward Left	Tso Lou Hsi Yao Pu
33.	海底撈針	Pick up the Needle from the Sea Bottom	Hai Ti Lao Chen
34.	扇通背	Fan Back	Shan T'ung Pei
35.	轉身撇身捶	Turn and Twist Body and Circle Fist	Chuan Shen Pieh Shen Ch'ui

36.	進步搬攔捶	Step Forward, Deflect Downward, Parry and Punch	Chin Pu, Pan, Lan Ch'ui
37.	上步掤攦擠按	Step Forward, Ward-Off, Rollback, Press and Push	Shang Pu, P'eng, Lu, Ghi, An
38.	單鞭	Single Whip	Tan Pien
39.	右雲手	Wave Hands in the Clouds: Right	Yu Yun Shou
40.	左雲手	Wave Hands in the Clouds: Left	Tso Yun Shou
41.	右雲手	Wave Hands in the Clouds: Right	Yu Yun Shou
42.	單鞭	Single Whip	Tan Pien
43.	高探馬	Stand High to Search Out the Horse	Kao T'an Ma
44.	右分脚	Separate Right Foot	Yu Fen Chiao
45.	左分脚	Separate Left Foot	Tso Fen Chiao
46.	轉身蹬脚	Turn and Kick with Heel (90 degrees)	Chuan Shen Teng Chiao
47.	左摟膝拗步	Brush Knee and Step Forward: Left	Tso Lou Hsi Yao Pu
48.	右摟膝拗步	Brush Knee and Step Forward: Right	Yu Lou Hsi Yao Pu
49.	進步栽捶	Step Forward and Strike Down with the Fist	Chin Pu Tsai Ch'ui
50.	轉身撇身捶	Turn and Twist the Body and Circle the Arm	Chuan Shen Pieh Shen Ch'ui
51.	進步搬攔捶	Step Forward, Deflect Downward, Parry and Punch	Chin Pu, Pan, Lan, Ch'ui
52.	右踢脚	Kick Right	Yu Ti Chiao
53.	右打虎	Strike the Tiger: Right	Yu Ta Fu
54.	左打虎	Strike the Tiger: Left	Tso Ta Fu
55.	右踢脚	Kick Right	Yu Ti Chiao
56.	双風貫耳	Attack the Ears by Fists	Shuang Feng Kuan Erh
57.	左踢脚	Kick Left	Tso Ti Chiao
58.	轉身蹬脚	Turn and Kick with Heel (270 degrees)	Chuan Shen Teng Chiao
59.	撇身捶	Twist Body and Circle Hands	Pieh Shen Ch'ui
60.	進步搬攔捶	Step Forward, Deflect Downward, Parry and Punch	Chin Pu Pan Lan Ch'ui
61.	如封似閉	Seal Tightly	Ju Feng Ssu Pi
62.	抱虎歸山	Embrace Tiger and Return to the Mountain	Pao Hu Guei Shan
63.	合太極	Close Tai Chi	Ho T'ai-Chi
64.	掤攦擠按	Ward-Off, Rollback, Press and Push	Peng, Lu, Ghi, An
65.	單鞭	Single Whip	Tan Pien
66.	右野馬分鬃	Wild Horses Share Mane: Right	Yu Yeh Ma Fen Tsung
67.	左野馬分鬃	Wild Horses Share Mane: Left	Tso Yeh Ma Fen Tsung
68.	右野馬分鬃	Wild Horses Share Mane: Right	Yu Yeh Ma Fen Tsung
69.	左攬雀尾	Grasp Sparrow's Tail: Left	Tso Lan Ch'iao Wei
70.	掤攦擠按	Ward-Off, Rollback, Press and Push	Peng, Lu, Ghi, An
71.	單鞭	Single Whip	Tan Pien
72.	左玉女穿梭	Fair Lady Weaves Shuttle: Left	Tso Yu Nu Ch'uan Suo
73.	右玉女穿梭	Fair Lady Weaves Shuttle: Right	Yu Yu Nu Ch'uan Suo
74.	左玉女穿梭	Fair Lady Weaves Shuttle: Left	Tso Yu Nu Ch'uan Suo
75.	右玉女穿梭	Fair Lady Weaves Shuttle: Right	Yu Yu Nu Ch'uan Suo
76.	左攬雀尾	Grasp Sparrow's Tail: (Left)	Tso Lan Ch'iao Wei
77. (4-7)	掤攦擠按	Ward-Off, Rollback, Press and Push	Peng, Lu, Ghi, An

78.	單鞭	Single Whip	Tan Pien
79.	右雲手	Wave Hands in Clouds: Right	Yu Yun Shou
80.	單鞭	Single Whip	Tan Pien
81.	蛇身下勢	Lower the Snake Body	Shr Shen Hsia Shih
82.	右金雞獨立	Golden Rooster Stands by One Leg: Right	Yu Chin Chi Tu Li
83.	左金雞獨立	Golden Rooster Stands by One Leg: Left	Tso Chin Chi Tu Li
84.	左倒攆猴	Step Back and Repulse Monkey: Left	Tso Tao Nien Hou
85.	斜飛勢	Diagonal Flying	Hsieh Fei Shih
86.	提手上勢	Left Hands and Lean Forward	T'i Shou Shang Shih
87.	白鶴亮翅	Crane Spreads Its Wings	Pai Hao Liang Ch'ih
88.	左摟膝拗步	Brush Knee and Step Forward: Left	Tso Lou Hsi Yao Pu
89.	海底撈針	Pick up the Needle from the Sea Bottom	Hai Ti Lao Chen
90.	扇通背	Fan Back	Shan T'ung Pei
91.	轉身白蛇吐信	White Snake Turns Body and Spits Poison	Chuan Shen Pai She T'u Hsin
92.	進步搬攔捶	Step Forward, Deflect Downward Parry and Punch	Chin Pu Pan Lan Ch'ui
93.	上步掤攦擠按	Step Forward, Ward-Off, Rollback, Press and Push	Shang Pu Peng, Lu, Ghi, An
94.	單鞭	Single Whip	Tan Pien
95.	右雲手	Wave Hands in Clouds: Right	Yu Yun Shou
96.	單鞭	Single Whip	Tan Pien
97.	高探馬	Stand High to Search Out the Horse	Kao T'an Ma
98.	十字手	Cross Hands	Shih Tzu Shou
99.	轉身十字腿	Turn and Kick	Chuan Shen Shih Tzu T'ui
100.	摟膝指襠捶	Brush Knee and Punch Down	Lou Hsi Chih Tang Ch'ui
101.	上步掤攦擠按	Step Forward, Ward-Off, Rollback, Press and Push	Shang Pu P'eng Lu, Ghi, An
102.	單鞭	Single Whip	Tan Pien
103.	蛇身下勢	Lower the Snake Body	Shr Shen Hsia Shih
104.	上步七星	Step Forward to Seven Stars	Shang Pu Ch'i Hsing
105.	退步跨虎	Step Back and Ride the Tiger	T'ui Pu K'ua Fu
106.	轉身擺蓮	Turn Body and Sweep Lotus with Leg	Chuan Shen Pai Lien
107.	彎弓射虎	Draw the Bow and Shoot the Tiger	Wan Kung She Fu
108.	撇身捶	Twist Body and Circle Hand	Pieh Shen Ch'ui
109.	進步搬攔捶	Step Forward, Deflect Downward, Parry and Punch	Chin Pu Pan Lan Ch'ui
110.	如封似閉	Seal Tightly	Ju Feng Ssu Pi
111.	抱虎歸山	Embrace the Riger and Return to the Mountain	Pao Hu Guei Shan
112.	合太極	Close Tai Chi	Ho T'ai-Chi
113.	太極還原	Return to the Original Stance	T'ai-Chi Huan Yuan

YANG'S TAI CHI SWORD

No.	Chinese	English	Pronunciation
1.	起勢	Beginning	Ch'i Shih
2.	上步合劍	Step Forward and Close With Sword	Shang Pu Ho Chien Shih
3.	仙人指路	Fairy Shows The Way	Hsien Jen Chih Lu
4.	三環套月	Three Rings Envelope the Moon	San Fuan T'ao Yueh
5.	大魁星	Big Chief Star	Da Kuai Hsing
6.	燕子抄水	Swallow Seizes Water	Yen Tzu Ch'ao Shui
7.	左右攔掃	Left Sweep: Right Sweep	Tso Yu Lan Sao
8.	小魁星	Little Chief Star	Hsiao Kuai Hsing
9.	黃蜂入洞	Yellow Bee Enters the Hole	Huang Fong Zoo Don
10.	靈貓捕鼠	Spirit Cat Catches the Mouse	Ling Mao Pu Su
11.	蜻蜓點水	Dragonfly Touches Water	Ching T'ing Tien Shui
12.	燕子入巢	Swallow Enters the Nest	Yen Tzu Zoo Ch'ao
13.	鳳凰双辰翅	Phoenix Spreads Its Wings	Fong Huang Shuang Chan Ch'ih
14.	右旋風	Right Whirlwind	Yu Shuen Fong
15.	小魁星	Little Chief Star	Hsiao Kuai Hsing
16.	左旋風	Left Whirlwind	Tso Shuen Fong
17.	等魚式	Wait For the Fish	Teng Yu Shih
18.	撥草尋蛇	Open Grass In Search of Snake	Poa Ts'ao Shoon Sir
19.	懷中抱月	Hold the Moon Against the Chest	Fuai Chung Pao Yueh
20.	送鳥上林	Send Bird to the Woods	Song Niao Shang Lin
21.	烏龍擺尾	Black Dragon Waves Its Tail	Wu Long Bai Wei
22.	風捲荷葉	Wind Blows the Lotus Leaf	Fong Chuan Ho Yeh
23.	獅子搖頭	Lion Shakes Its Head	Shih Tzu Yao T'ou
24.	虎抱頭	Tiger Holds Its Head	Fu Pao T'ou
25.	野馬跳澗	Wild Horse Jumps the Stream	Yeh Ma T'iao Jen
26.	翻身勒馬	Turn Body and Rein In Horse	Fan Shen Duh Ma
27.	指南針	Compass	Chih Nan Chen
28.	迎風撣塵	Clean Up Dust In the Wind	Ying Fong Tan Ch'en
29.	順手推舟	Push Boat With the Current	Shun Shui T'uai Chou
30.	流星趕月	Shooting Star Chasing the Moon	Lieo Hsing Kan Yueh
31.	天鳥飛瀑	Bird Flying Over the Water Fall	T'ien Niao Fei P'u
32.	挑簾勢	Raise the Screen	T'iao Lien Shih
33.	左右車輪劍	Left and Right Wheel Sword	Tso Yu Ch'e Lun Chien
34.	燕子啣泥	Swallow Picks Up Mud With Beak	Yen Tzu Shen Ni
35.	大鵬展翅	A Roc Spreads Its Wing	Ta P'eng Chan Ch'ih
36.	海底撈月	Pick Up the Moon From the Sea Bottom	Hai Ti Lao Yueh
37.	懷中抱月	Hold the Moon Against the Chest	Fuai Chung Pao Yueh
38.	夜叉探海	Night Demon Gauges the Depth of the Sea	Yeh Ch'a T'an Hai
39.	犀牛望月	A Rhino Looks at the Moon	Hsi Nieu Wang Yueh
40.	射雁勢	Shoot the Geese	Sheh Yen Shih
41.	青龍探爪	Blue Dragon Waves His Claws	Ch'ing Long T'an Jwa
42;	凤凰双辰翅	Phoenix Spreads His Wings	Fong Huang Shuang Chan Ch'ih
43.	左右跨攔	Left and Right Step Over Obstacle	Tso Yu K'ua Lan
44.	射雁勢	Shoot the Geese	Sheh Yen Shih

45.	白猿献果	White Ape Offers Up Fruit	Pai Yuen Hsien Guoo
46.	落花势	Falling Flowers Posture	Loa Fua Shih
47.	玉女穿梭	Fair Lady Weaves Shuttle	Yu Nu Ch'uan Suo
48.	白虎攬尾	White Tiger Waves Its Tail	Pai Fu Chow Wei
49.	魚跳龍門	Fish Jump Into Dragon Gate	Yu T'iao Long Mun
50.	烏龍絞柱	Black Dragon Wraps Around Post	Wu Long Chow Tsuh
51.	仙人指路	Fairy Shows the Way: Second Form	Hsien Jen Chih Lu
52.	風掃梅花	Wind Blows Away the Plum Flowers	Fong Sao Mei Fua
53.	手捧牙笏	To Hold A Tablet	Shou P'eng Ya Fu
54.	扼劍歸原	Hold the Sword and Return to Original Stance	Pao Jen Kuai Yuan

ABOUT THE AUTHOR

Dr. Yang Jwing-Ming started his training in Yang's style of Tai Chi Chuan in 1962, at the age of sixteen, with Master Kao Taou. Master Kao Taou himself learned Tai Chi Chuan from his father. Dr. Yang started Tai Chi on the advice of his Shao Lin White Crane master, Cheng Gin-Gsao, as a possible remedy for stomach problems. Dr. Yang studied Tai Chi with Master Kao Taou for almost three years, during which time Dr. Yang mastered the barehand sequence (105 forms) and pushing hands. Through the practice of Tai Chi, the author experienced its healthful benefits; he cured his stomach ailment and, unexpectedly, also relieved his sinus problems.

When Dr. Yang began his schooling in Taipei in 1964, he continued to further his research and improve his abilities in Yang's style of Tai Chi with the Shao Lin Long Fist Master Li Mao-Ching. Master Li Mao-Ching learned Yang's Tai Chi from Master Han Ching-Tan of the Central Kuo Su Institute; Master Han himself learned Yang's Tai Chi from the famous grandson of the founder, Yang Chen-Fu.

During the early 1970s, Dr. Yang continued his study of Tai Chi by researching Yang's style with Chen Wei-Shen. Chen Wei-Shen had previously studied Tai Chi with Master Chang Shian-Shan. Both Chen and the author combined their skills and knowledge to greatly enhance their overall mastery. Their research took in many areas, especially Tai Chi free fighting.

After coming to America in 1974 to study for his Ph.D. in mechanical engineering at Purdue University, Dr. Yang continued to study, practice, and research Tai Chi on his own. While at Purdue, besides receiving his Ph.D., the author taught credited coruses in Tai Chi for over five years. This experience is in addition to his seven years of teaching Tai Chi in Taiwan.

Overall, Dr. Yang has mastered the barehand sequence, pushing hands, the two-man fighting sequence, narrow and wide blade sword, and internal power development. These skills were learned and practiced over an eighteen-year period of research with various masters and Tai Chi students.

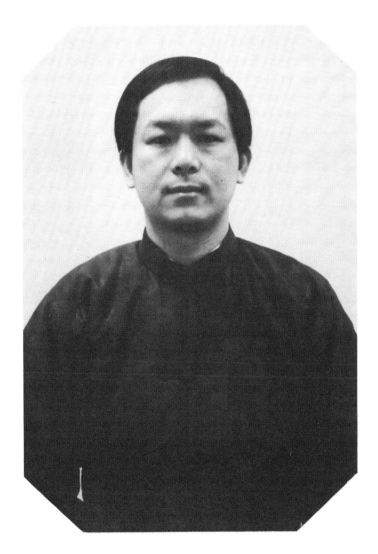

Master Yang Jwing-Ming